Second Edition

Insulin in Clinical Practice

Second Edition

Insulin in Clinical Practice

Manthappa M MD (Medicine)
Professor
Department of Medicine and
Vice Principal, JSS Medical College
JSS Academy of Higher Education and Research
Mysore, Karnataka

Former Associate Professor, Department of Medicine
Kasturba Medical College, Manipal University (now MAHE)
Manipal, Karnataka

Email: manthappa@yahoo.com

CBSPD

CBS Publishers & Distributors Pvt Ltd

New Delhi • Bengaluru • Chennai • Kochi • Kolkata • Lucknow • Mumbai
Gujarat • Hyderabad • Jharkhand • Nagpur • Patna • Pune • Uttarakhand

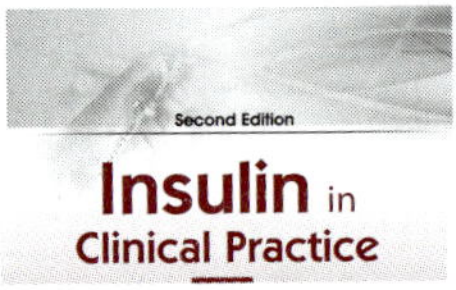

ISBN: 978-93-5466-599-8

Second Edition: 2024

Reprint: **2025**

Published by **Satish Kumar Jain** and produced by **Varun Jain** for

CBS Publishers & Distributors Pvt Ltd

4819/XI Prahlad Street, 24 Ansari Road, Daryaganj, New Delhi 110 002, India
Ph: 011-23289259, 23266838 Website: www.cbspd.com
e-mail: delhi@cbspd.com

Corporate Office: 204 FIE, Industrial Area, Patparganj, Delhi 110 092, India
Ph: 011-49344934 Fax: 011-49344935 e-mail: publishing@cbspd.com; publicity@cbspd.com

Branches

- **Bengaluru:** Seema House 2975, 17th Cross, K.R. Road, Banasankari 2nd Stage, Bengaluru 560 070, Karnataka, India
  Ph: +91-80-26771678/79 Fax: +91-80-26771680 e-mail: bangalore@cbspd.com
- **Chennai:** 18/8B, Subbaraya Street, Shenoy Nagar, Chennai 600 030, Tamil Nadu, India
  Ph: +91-44-26680620, 26681266 e-mail: chennai@cbspd.com
- **Kochi:** 42/1325, 1326, Power House Road, Opposite KSEB, Power House, Ernakulum 682018, Kochi, Kerala, India
  Ph: +91-484-4059061–65 Fax: +91-484-4059065 e-mail: kochi@cbspd.com
- **Kolkata:** 147, Hind Ceramics Compound, 1st Floor, Nilgunj Road, Belghoria, Kolkata 700056, West Bengal, India
  Ph: +91-33-25330055/56 e-mail: kolkata@cbspd.com
- **Lucknow:** Basement, Khushuma Complex, 7 Meerabai Marg (behind Jawahar Bhawan), Lucknow 226001, UP, India
  Ph: +91-522-4000032 e-mail: tiwari.lucknow@cbspd.com
- **Mumbai:** PWD Shed, Gala No. 25/26, Ramchandra Bhatt Marg, Next JJ Hospital, Gate No. 2, Opp. Union Bank of India, Noorbaug, Mumbai 400009, Maharashtra, India
  Ph: +91-22-66661880/89 e-mail: mumbai@cbspd.com

Representatives

- **Gujarat** 0-9879558667
- **Hyderabad** 0-9885175004
- **Jharkhand** 0-9811541605
- **Nagpur** 0-8692091830
- **Patna** 0-9334159340
- **Pune** 0-9664372571
- **Uttarakhand** 0-9716462459

Printed at Sri Print and Sales, Delhi, India

to

my brother

MK Swamy

who has been a constant source of

courage, support, and inspiration to me

Preface to the Second Edition

I am very happy to place before you the second edition of the book *Insulin in Clinical Practice*. All the latest literature about insulin and various insulin regimens has been referred to make this second edition up-to-date and more useful to clinicians.

The discovery of insulin has been one of the greatest milestones in medicine. In fact, the discoverers got Nobel Prize for this achievement in medicine. We can control any type of diabetes mellitus by using insulin. When all the oral anti-diabetic drugs fail to work, insulin is the savior and always works. Type 1 diabetes requires insulin from the beginning of diagnosis and type 2 diabetes requires it at some point of time either temporarily or permanently. Gestational diabetes and other secondary types of diabetes also require insulin. With the availability of many types of insulins, managing diabetes is far more easier now than before, and treatment can be tailored to individual needs. But using insulin is not easy. Its rational and effective use requires common sense, intelligence, and sound knowledge of different types of insulins, their time–action profiles and different insulin regimens. Everyone is familiar with insulin but a few are real experts in using it. Literature is scattered in different sources when it comes to using insulin. Here I have made sincere efforts to bring together all the available data about insulin in a simple language.

This book is useful for all the general practitioners, post-graduate students, residents, physicians, and all other doctors who are engaged in treating diabetes mellitus. The purpose of this book is to make you an expert in using insulin.

Manthappa M

Contents

Chapter

1

Diagnosis of Diabetes Mellitus

Diabetes mellitus is a major disease which is increasing in the world day-by-day. Uncontrolled diabetes can lead to blindness, limb amputation, kidney failure, and vascular and heart disease. It is a silent disease and can cause lot of complications mentioned above if not diagnosed early. To diagnose diabetes mellitus early, all adults without risk factors should be screened with a test for prediabetes and type 2 diabetes starting at age 35. All women who are planning to become pregnant should be screened for diabetes by doing a fasting glucose test, especially if they have risk factors. For unplanned pregnancies, women should be screened at the first prenatal visit. Screening for gestational diabetes should be done again between 24 and 28 weeks.

ADA (American Diabetes Association) Criteria to Diagnose Diabetes Mellitus:

Diabetes is diagnosed with any one of the following criteria:	
1.	FBS ≥ 126 mg/dL, fasting is defined as no caloric intake for at least 8 hours OR
2.	2 hours post load glucose ≥ 200 mg/dL during an OGTT(oral glucose tolerance test). The test should be performed as described by WHO, using a glucose load containing the equivalent of 75 g anhydrous glucose dissolved in water OR
3.	A1C ≥ 6.5% OR
4.	Random plasma glucose ≥ 200 mg/dL in a patient with classic symptoms of hyperglycemia or hyperglycemic crisis. Random is defined as anytime of the day without regard to time since last meal. The classic symptoms of diabetes include polyuria, polydypsia, and unexplained weight loss

The above tests should be repeated once more to confirm the presence of diabetes mellitus unless there is a clear clinical diagnosis (e.g., patient in a hyperglycemic crisis or with classic symptoms of hyperglycemia and a random plasma glucose ≥ 200 mg/dL). Second test should be done as early as possible without much delay.

OGTT should be performed under controlled conditions to ensure its accuracy. Factors that decrease the value of OGTT include:

1. Carbohydrate restriction (<150 gm for 3 days)
2. Bed rest or severe inactivity
3. Medical or surgical stress
4. Drugs (e.g. Thiazides, steroids, β-blockers, phenytoin)
5. Smoking
6. Anxiety from repeated needle sticks.

Hence, OGTT should not be performed in acutely ill patients. Patients should ideally stop smoking and consume a liberal carbohydrate meal for at least 3 days prior to testing.

CRITERIA TO DIAGNOSE PREDIABETES STATES

"Prediabetes" is the term used for individuals whose glucose levels do not meet the criteria for diabetes but have glucose levels more than the cut-off for normal individuals. These people have abnormal carbohydrate metabolism and are at risk of developing diabetes in future. Prediabetes is diagnosed by the presence of any one of the following criteria.

Impaired fasting glucose (IFG)
Fasting plasma glucose (FPG) 100 mg/dL to 125 mg/dL OR
Impaired glucose tolerance (IGT)
2 h plasma glucoe during 75 g OGTT 140 mg/dL to 199 mg/dL OR
A1C 5.7–6.4%

All patients with prediabetes states should be treated with diet and exercise and should be followed up yearly for the progression to diabetes.

Classification of Diabetes Mellitus

The ADA classification of diabetes includes four clinical classes:

- Type 1 diabetes (results from β-cell destruction, usually leading to absolute insulin deficiency).
- Type 2 diabetes (results from a progressive insulin secretory defect on the background of insulin resistance).
- Other specific types of diabetes due to other causes, e.g., genetic defects in β-cell function, genetic defects in insulin action, diseases of the exocrine pancreas (such as cystic fibrosis), and drug or chemical induced (such as in the treatment of AIDS or after organ transplantation).
- Gestational diabetes mellitus (GDM) (diagnosed during pregnancy).

How to Know the Type of Diabetes

Understanding the type of diabetes is important from treatment point of view. However, many people do not fit exactly into one type. For example, some people with type 1 diabetes may become obese and develop insulin resistance which is a feature of type 2 diabetes. On the other hand most type 2 diabetics in advanced stages have little or no endogenous insulin secretion and such people have the characteristics of type 1 diabetes. Blurring of the lines between type 1 and type 2 diabetes is increasingly becoming common.

Clinical Clues

Type 1 diabetes usually begins in childhood, but can occur at any age. Approximately 50% of the adults develop type 1 diabetes before the age 40 years. The remainders develop it as older adults. Presence of other autoimmune diseases like celiac disease, Graves' disease, hypothyroidism, Addisons disease, pernicious anemia, etc. suggests type 1 diabetes. Family history of type 1 diabetes again suggests type 1 diabetes in the patient. Persons with type 1 diabetes are usually thin and have very high blood sugars at presentation. They often present with diabetic ketoacidosis. A type 2 diabetic is usually obese, presents after 35 years of age and may satisfy the criteria of metabolic syndrome. If the person is on oral antidiabetic agents and is controlled with it, then he has type 2 diabetes because obviously oral agents do not work in type 1 diabetes.

Laboratory Clues

Ketone bodies: Presence of a large amount of ketone bodies goes in favour of type 1 diabetes, though type 2 also can have ketone bodies. If insulin is injected before testing for ketone bodies, the opportunity to find a large amounts of ketone bodies may be missed.

C- peptide levels: C-peptide is half of the precursor molecule to insulin that is split off when insulin is produced from the body. C-peptide levels can reveal how much insulin a person is producing. If c-peptide level is normal or high, type 2 diabetes is likely. If significantly low type 1 diabetes is likely. If the level is low normal, the person may have early type 1 or longstanding type 2 DM. When external insulin is being used it may suppress endogenous insulin production and hence c-peptide levels may be low. C-peptide levels should be measured after insulin has been reduced or discontinued, and the blood sugar has risen to 200 mg/dL or more.

Antibodies: Type 1 diabetes is an autoimmune disease, hence anti-islet anti-bodies and anti-GAD 65 (glutamic acid decorboxylase) antibodies can be found in 80 – 90% of patients with type 1 diabetes. Anti-GAD 65 antibodies can be found in only 3% of normal population. When both islet cell and GAD 65 antibodies are detected they increase the autoimmune disease detection to >90%. Blood tests can be done to detect the presence of these antibodies. If the person does not already have diabetes, presence of these antibodies predicts development of type 1 diabetes in such persons.

High triglyceride, low HDL, high uric acid: All these are markers of metabolic syndrome and suggest type 2 diabetes.

Glucose clamp procedure to detect insulin resistance: This is the gold standard to detect insulin resistance. Insulin resistance suggests type 2 diabetes. However, this is a time consuming procedure and is used only in research settings.

All the above lab tests especially C-peptide levels and auto antibodies need not be done routinely. Use them only when a person's diabetes type is not clear or when treatment is not working for unknown reasons.

Glycemic Targets for Adults with Diabetes as per American Diabetes Association (ADA):

A1C	***< 7.0%***
Preprandial capillary plasma glucose	80 – 130 mg/dL (4.4 to 7.2 mmol/l)
Peak postprandial capillary plasma glucose	< 180 mg/dL (< 10.0 mmol/l)

Blood Pressure Targets

For individuals with diabetes and hypertension at higher CV risk, a blood pressure target of <130/80 mmHg may be appropriate, if it can be safely attained.

For individuals with diabetes and hypertension at lower risk for CVD a target blood pressure of <140/90 mmHg is acceptable.

Lipid Targets

2018 AHA/ACC/Guideline on the management of blood cholesterol recommends treatment with a statin for 4 groups of patients, comprised of those with any of the following:

- Clinical ASCVD (atherosclerotic cardiovascular disease)
- LDL cholesterol ≥ 190 mg/dL
- Age 40 to 75, with diabetes and LDL cholesterol 70 to 189 mg/dL
- Age 40 to 75, LDL cholesterol 70 to 189 mg/dL, and estimated 10-year risk of ASCVD ≥ 7.5%

For primary prevention, statin therapy should lower LDL-C approximately 30% to more than 50%.

For secondary prevention, as defined by a patient who has coronary artery disease, a target goal is set for LDL-C less than 70 mg/dL.

If the patient is a high risk (already had acute coronary syndrome in the last year, familial hypercholesterolemia, diabetes, chronic kidney disease (stage 3 or 4), or atherosclerotic cardiovascular disease event, or the need for revascularization while on a statin), then the LDL goal should be less than 50.

A1C Level

- A1C is the primary tool for assessing glycemic control and has a strong predictive value for diabetes complications. The A1C goal *for patients in general* is <7%. TheA1C goal *for the individual patient* is as close to normal (<6%) as possible without significant hypoglycemia.
- An A1C goal for many nonpregnant adults of <7% (53 mmol/mol) without significant hypoglycemia is appropriate.
- On the basis of provider judgment and patient preference, achievement of lower A1C levels than the goal of 7% may be acceptable and even beneficial if it can be achieved safely without significant hypoglycemia or other adverse effects of treatment.
- Less stringent A1C goals (such as <8%) may be appropriate for patients with limited life expectancy or where the harms of treatment are greater than the benefits.
- Less stringent treatment goals may be appropriate for patients with a history of severe hypoglycemia, patients with limited life expectancy, very young children or older adults, and individuals with comorbid conditions.
- Aggressive glycemic management with insulin may reduce morbidity in patients with severe acute illness, perioperatively, following myocardial infarction, and in pregnancy.
- Goals should be individualized
- Postprandial glucose may be targeted if A1C goals are not met despite reaching preprandial glucose goals

A1C Testing Recommendations

- Perform the A1C test at least two times a year in patients who are meeting treatment goals (and who have stable glycemic control).
- Perform the A1C test once in 3 months in patients whose therapy has changed or who are not meeting glycemic goals.
- Use of point-of-care testing for A1C allows for timely decision on therapy changes, when needed.

Chapter

2

Insulin Basics

Discovery of insulin was one of the greatest milestones in medicine. It was discovered in 1921 by Banting and Best and they tried this on a patient in 1922. They received Nobel Prize in medicine for this remarkable discovery. The structure of insulin was subsequently fully worked out by Sanger in 1956.

DISULFIDE BONDS

Insulin is a two-chain polypeptide having 51 amino acids and molecular wt of 6000. These two polypeptide chains have been named as A and B chains **(Fig. 2.1)**. A chain contains 21 amino acids and B chain contains 30 amino acids. The A and B chains are held together by disulfide bonds. Insulin from different species differs only by a few amino acids. There are only minor differences between human, pork and beef insulins **(Table 2.1)**.

Note that the pork insulin resembles human insulin more than beef insulin. Pork insulin differs from human insulin by only one amino acid, whereas beef insulin differs by three amino acids.

Insulins of bovine or porcine origin were the only commercially available preparations for the first half century

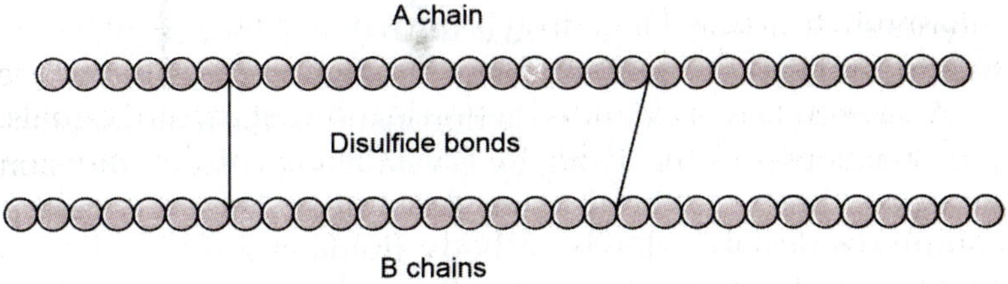

Fig. 2.1: Structure of insulin

Table 2.1: Differences in the amino acid composition of human, pork and beef insulin

Species	***A chain***	***B chain***	
	8th AA	10th AA	30th AA
Human	THR	ILEU	THR
Pork (porcine)	THR	ILEU	ALA
Beef (bovine)	ALA	VAL	ALA

of the insulin era. Though animal insulins differ slightly from human insulin as explained above, they are reliably absorbed into the human systemic circulation after subcutaneous injection and provide good control of plasma glucose. Limitations are mainly due to allergic reactions to impurities present in the formulations or the insulin molecule itself.

The first commercially available beef and pork insulins were amorphous solutions produced by alcohol extraction and acid precipitation. The addition of trace amounts of zinc to this process resulted in the formation of insulin crystals and production of the first short acting (crystalline zinc) insulin. This was called regular insulin or plain insulin. This had a short duration of action (5 – 8 hr).

The duration of action of subcutaneously injected insulin was further prolonged by complexing with protamine, a protein of fish origin. The protamine insulin complex is poorly soluble at physiologic pH and thus slowly absorbed from the subcutaneous tissue. Addition of trace amounts of zinc and further improvement in the molecule resulted in neutral protamine hagedron (NPH or isophane) insulin, which is intermediate acting. Hagedron is the name of the scientist who first formulated this preparation.

A second class of extended action insulins, the lente insulins, was developed in the 1950s by crystallizing insulin and zinc in acetate buffer without using protamine. These crystalline complexes dissolve slowly in body fluids and thus exhibit a prolonged duration of action after subcutaneous injection. Two types of insulins resulted by this method, semilente and ultralente. Semilente has a peak and duration of action slightly longer than regular insulin. Ultralente has the greatest stability, lowest peak and long duration of action. Combining semilente and ultralente in the ratio of 30% and 70% gives lente insulin, which has a time action profile similar to NPH. Semilente is not used now except for producing lente.

So now we have NPH, lente and ultralente insulins. NPH and lente are intermediate acting and ultralente is long-acting. However, lente, semilente, and ultralente insulins are not available now.

HUMAN INSULIN

Refinement of microbiologic techniques led to the production of biosynthetic human insulin in 1980s. The first commercially available preparations of human insulin were sold from 1982 onwards. Recombinant human insulin is produced predominantly using *E. coli* and *Saccharomyces cerevisiae* for therapeutic use in human. In future, plant-based expression system hold tremendous potential for high-capacity production of insulin in very cost-effective manner. Very high level of expression of biologically active proinsulin in seeds or leaves with long-term stability, offers a low-cost technology for both injectable as well as oral delivery of proinsulin.

How to Measure Insulin Levels

1 mg of the international standard of insulin is 24 units. Insulin can be bioassayed by measuring blood sugar in rabbits or by its potency to induce hypoglycemic convulsions in mice. As pure preparations are now available, it can be assayed chemically also. Plasma insulin can be measured by radio immunoassay or enzyme immunoassay.

Regulation of Insulin Secretion

Insulin is secreted by beta-cells of pancreas. Under basal conditions, 1 unit insulin is secreted per hour by human pancreas. A larger quantity than this is secreted after every meal. Insulin secretion from beta-cells is regulated by chemical, hormonal, and neural mechanisms.

Chemical Control

Glucose, amino acids, fatty acids, and ketone bodies can stimulate insulin release, but glucose is the most powerful stimulus among these. Glucose and other nutrients are more effective in stimulating insulin release when given orally than intravenously because of generation of chemical signals (incretins) from the gut, which act on beta cells to cause anticipatory release of insulin. The incretins involved are gut-glucagon, secretin, gastrin, gastric inhibitory polypeptide, VIP, cholecystokinin – pancreozymin, etc.

Hormonal Control

GH, corticosteroids, thyroxine, prostaglandins, etc. have influence on insulin secretion. Different Islet cells of pancreas (alpha, beta, and delta) have influence on each other (paracrine effect).

Somatostatin (from delta cells), inhibits the release of both insulin and glucagon **(Fig. 2.2)**.

Glucagon (from alpha cells) evokes release of insulin as well as somatostatin.

Insulin (from beta cells) inhibits glucagon secretion.

Neural Control

The islets are richly supplied by sympathetic and parasympathetic (vagus) nerves.

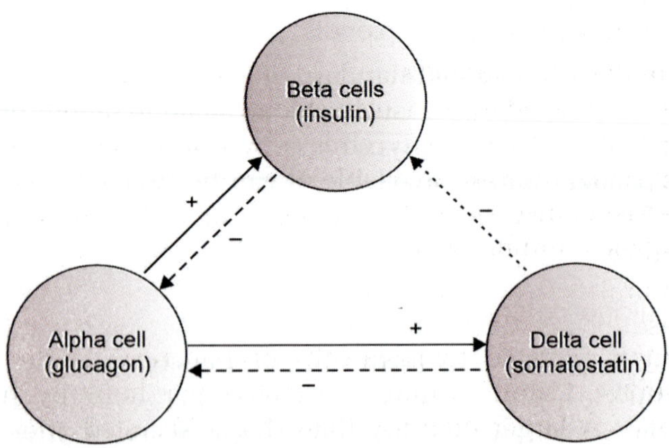

Fig. 2.2: Hormonal control of insulin secretion

Sympathetic

Adrenergic alpha-2 receptor activation inhibits insulin release by inhibiting beta-cell adenyl cyclase (prominent action). Adrenergic beta-2 stimulation increases insulin release by stimulating beta cell adenyl cyclase (less prominent action).

Parasympathetic

Muscarinic activation by acetylcholine or vagal stimulation causes increased insulin secretion.

Hypothalamus

Stimulation of ventrolateral nucleus in hypothalamus evokes insulin release, whereas stimulation of ventromedial nuclei inhibits insulin release.

Actions of Insulin

The ultimate goal of insulin is to favour storage of fuel:

- It facilitates glucose transport across cell membranes. Skeletal muscle and fat are highly sensitive to this action. However, glucose entry into liver, brain, RBC, WBC and renal medullary cells is largely independent of insulin. Muscular activity induces glucose entry into muscle cells without the need for insulin, hence exercise has insulin sparing effect.
- It inhibits glycogenolysis in liver and facilitates glycogen synthesis (by stimulating glycogen synthetase) in liver, muscle, and fat.
- It inhibits gluconeogenesis (from protein) in liver and thus has protein sparing effect.
- It inhibits lipolysis in adipose tissue and favors triglyceride synthesis
- It stimulates transcription of vascular endothelial lipoprotein lipase and thus increases clearance of VLDL and chylomicrons.
- It facilitates amino acid entry and their synthesis into proteins in muscle cells and possibly other cells. Insulin deficiency leads to protein breakdown. In the absence of insulin, catabolism takes the upper hand over anabolism and this is what happens in diabetes.

Mechanism of Action

Insulin acts on specific receptors located on cell membranes of practically all tissues, but the density of receptors is highest in liver and fat cells. Each receptor consists of four total units (two alpha and two beta). The alpha sub units bind to insulin and beta sub units have tyrosine kinase activity. When insulin binds to its receptor, the receptor and insulin complex is internalized and a series of phosphorylation and dephosphorylation reactions are set into motion which ultimately result in the appropriate action of insulin **(Table 2.2)**.

Table 2.2: Factors affecting the bioavailability and absorption rate of subcutaneously injected insulin

Factor	*Effect*
Type of insulin	Human insulin is more rapidly absorbed than animal insulin. Aspart and lispro are more rapidly absorbed than regular insulin. Glargine is absorbed very slowly
Site of injection	Abdominal injection results in more rapid absorption than thigh or arm
Depth of injection	IM injections are more rapidly absorbed than SC injections
Insulin concentration	Dilute solutions (U 40) are absorbed more rapidly than concentrated solutions (U 100)
Dose of insulin	Higher doses of injected insulin have more prolonged action than lower doses
Mixing insulins	Regular insulin maintains its potency and time-action profile when mixed with NPH insulin, but mixing with lente or ulterlente significantly slows absorption and blunts the activity of regular insulin
Exercise	Exercising a muscle group prior to injection into that area increases the rate of insulin absorption because of increased blood supply
Local heat, massage	Local heat and massage following injection increases the rate of absorption of insulin due to increased blood supply

Insulin stimulates glucose transport across cell membrane by ATP dependent dislocation of glucose transporters to the plasma membrane as well as by increasing their activity. It is also needed for the expression of the genes responsible for the synthesis of the glucose transporters.

New insulin preparations like glargine and detemir are not much affected by these factors.

Fate of Insulin

Since insulin is a polypeptide, it is degraded in GIT if given orally. Injected insulin or that released from pancreas is distributed only extracellularly and is metabolized mainly in liver and to a lesser extent in kidney and muscles. Hence in liver failure plasma insulin concentration may become high and cause hypoglycemia. Degradation of insulin after receptor mediated internalization occurs to variable extent in most target cells. Insulin is ultimately broken down to its constituent amino acids. The plasma half life is about 5 to 9 minutes.

Insulin Concentrations Available in the Market

Insulin is commercially available in concentrations of 40, 100 or 500 units/mL (designated as U-40, U-100 and U-500). U-500 is only rarely used in cases of extreme insulin resistance, requiring large doses. Insulin preparations are sometimes formulated individually for use in infants (e.g. U-10) with diluents provided by the manufacturer.

Different types and species of insulin have different pharmacological properties. Human insulin is preferred for use in pregnant women, in individuals with allergies or antibodies to animal insulins, in those initiating therapy and those expected to use insulin only intermittently. All the animal insulins are slowly being phased out.

Since different species insulins have different pharmacokinetics, changing species may affect blood sugar control and should be done under medical supervision. Pharmacists and healthcare providers should not interchange insulin species or types without the approval of the prescribing doctor. If a patient is admitted to the hospital, the type of insulin he/she is using should not be changed unnecessarily. If there is doubt about which species insulin he was taking, human insulin should be administered until adequate information is available. In the event that a patient's particular brand of insulin is unavailable, the same type of insulin from a different manufacturer may be substituted. Changing insulin types (short, intermediate, etc.) should be done under medical supervision.

Storage of Insulin

Insulin should be kept in refrigerator, at a temperature between 2° and 3°C. It should not be freezed or exposed to higher temperatures.

Research has shown that if insulin is stored at room temperature, it loses 1.5% of its potency per month (after one month 1cc U-100 insulin would have 98.5 units of insulin rather than 100 units). For most people, this small change would not make a difference. It is preferable to discard bottles of insulin that have been opened for three or more months, even if kept in refrigerator. Insulin will spoil if it gets above 90°F or if it freezes. Insulin bottles (or pens) cannot be left in a car in the hot summer or the cold winter. If blood sugars rise, (for no other reason) after using the current insulin vials for longer than one month, replace them. Any other specific storage guidelines from the manufacturer have to be followed.

Injection of cold insulin into subcutaneous tissue sometimes causes local irritation. This is minimized by taking the vial out of refrigerator, well in advance of injection and allowing it to come to room temperature or alternatively the vial can be kept at room temperature for at least 1 month without loss of potency.

The solutions of insulin lispro, aspart, regular insulin, insulin glargine and insulin detemir are clear whereas NPH, lente, ultralente appear cloudy. Before injection the person injecting the insulin should inspect the vial for any change like clumping, frosting, precipitation, change in clarity or color. If so it should not be used. Whenever there is unexplained increase in blood glucose, the loss of potency of insulin should also be kept in mind. If there is any uncertainty about the potency of insulin, it should be replaced.

Mixing Insulins

When different types of insulins are mixed, physicochemical changes may occur either immediately or over time. As a result, physiological action of the mixture may be different than when they are injected separately.

Mixing of short acting insulin with intermediate or long-acting insulin reduces the number of injections. This has to be done just before the injection. However, now-a-days premixed insulins are widely available in the market and are very popular.

If mixing is being done before injection, patients should be instructed in the proper method of mixing insulins. In general, regular insulin should be drawn first into the syringe as this avoids the contamination of regular insulin vial with delayed action preparation which may prolong the action of regular insulin. Contamination of delayed-action-preparation vial with regular insulin does not have any effect on that preparation.

Mixing of short acting insulin with NPH (Neutral Protamine Hagedron) insulin does not alter the time-action profile of short-acting insulin since NPH insulin does not contain Zn ions. This has resulted in the development and marketing of many premixed insulin preparations of NPH and short acting insulins. Mixtures of regular and NPH are available in the concentrations of 70:30 and 50:50 (70% NPH and 30% regular) (50% NPH and 50% regular). Recently premixed preparations of neutral protamine lispro and lispro, neutral protamine aspart and aspart are available in the market. Though such insulin mix preparations limit the flexibility of insulin therapy, they are very useful in patients with impaired vision and impaired fine motor skills as most of the steps like measuring both insulins and drawing both into syringe are minimized.

Mixing of Insulins should Follow these Guidelines

- Patients well controlled with a particular mixed insulin regimen should maintain their standard procedure for preparing their insulin doses.
- No other medication or diluent should be mixed with any insulin product unless approved by the prescribing physician.

- Insulin glargine should not be mixed with any other insulin due to the low pH of its diluent. Eventhough some studies suggest that glargine can be mixed with short acting insulin immediately before injection, large trials are required to further clarify this.
- Commercially available premixed insulins may be used if the insulin ratio is appropriate to the patient's insulin requirements.
- Lispro insulin can be mixed with NPH, lente and ultratente (lente and ultralente not available now).
- When lispro insulin is mixed with either intermediate or long-acting insulin, the mixture should be injected within 15 minutes before a meal.
- Phosphate buffered insulins (e.g. NPH) should not be mixed with lente insulins.

Syringes

Insulin syringes are available as 0.3, 0.5, 1 and 2 mL capacities. 0.3 mL syringes are for insulin doses under 30 units of insulin and are numbered at 1-unit intervals.0.5 mL syringes are for 30 to 50 units of insulin and are numbered at 1-unit intervals. 1.0 mL are for doses more than 50 units of insulin and are numbered at 2 units per interval.

Needles are also available in different gauges and different lengths. Needle gauges (thickness) range from 28 to 31. Higher the gauge smaller is the thickness of needle. The BD Ultra-Fine needles are available in 31 gauge. Lengths of needles are available from 5 mm to 12.7 mm (half inch). The length of a needle determines how far into skin it penetrates. Needles for insulin only need to go into subcutaneous tissue and not into muscle. Shorter needles are safer to avoid going into the muscle. Small needles are helpful in young children. Manufacturers of disposable syringes and pen needles recommend a single use. One potential risk with reuse of syringes or needles is infection. If needle reuse is planned it should be recapped after every use. Certainly a needle should be discarded if it is visibly deformed or dull or if it has come into contact with any surface other than skin. The syringe also may be reused and it may be stored at room temperature. Cleaning the needle with alcohol is not desirable as it may remove the silicon coating on the needle that makes injections less painful. Jet injectors and pen devices, though costly offer many advantages to the patient.

Drawing Insulin into Syringe

- Always verify the label before injection
- Clean the injection site
- The insulin vial or pen should be gently rolled in the palm or shaken gently to resuspend the insulin. This is not necessary for short acting insulins, insulin glargine and insulin detemir as they are clear.
- An amount of air equal to the dose of insulin required should be injected into the vial to avoid creating a vacuum. For a mixed dose, put air into both bottles before drawing insulin.
- When mixing short-acting with long-acting insulin preparations prior to injection, the short acting insulin should be drawn up first in the syringe and then long-acting insulin. If you draw long-acting first and then put the syringe into short acting insulin vial, it may contaminate the short acting insulin vial and change the pharmacokinetics of short acting insulin. However, little contamination of long-acting insulin vial by short-acting isnulin does not have much effect.
- After the insulin is drawn into the syringe, remove air bubbles by few quick flicks of the forefinger against the upright syringe. Small air bubbles are not dangerous in themselves, but may decrease the dose of insulin injected.

Injection Techniques

Injections are given into the subcutaneous tissue. Clean the site of injection with soap and water or an alcohol swab. Lift the skin and fat tissue between the thumb and the first finger, and inject at 90° angle, if you are using short needles (5 mm and 6 mm) and the fat in the area of injection is adequate. 45° angle can be used for the half inch needles and for injection in thin individuals and children to avoid intramuscular injection. The needle should be in the subcutaneous tissue for at least 5 seconds if you are using pen device to ensure complete delivery of the insulin dose.

If there is not much fat, a gentle pinch should still be used during the injection. It is generally best to push the needle all the way into the skin. If the needle is not in far enough, the insulin may not be injected into the fatty layer. If it goes into the layer directly under the skin rather than into the fatty layer, it will sting and may cause a small swelling or redness and itching. If the needle is not close to the fingers holding the skin, the gentle pinch can continue to be held during the injection of the insulin. Inject the insulin by pushing the plunger down with a SLOW and steady push as far as it will go. Some people like to wait a few seconds to let the insulin "spread out" after each five units of insulin is injected. A smooth injection is important. After the insulin is in, wait five to ten seconds before removing the needle. This will help to prevent insulin leakage from the injection site. A loss of one drop of insulin may be equal to two to five units. Loss of insulin is a common reason for variations in the blood sugar levels. If "leak-back" continues to be a problem move to a new site. Also, two units of air can be drawn into the syringe after removing the needle from the insulin bottle. Then flick the side of the syringe with a finger to make the air rise up under the plunger. The air will then be injected after the insulin and will help to prevent"leak-back."

After the injection, place a finger or dry cotton swab over the site of injection. Hold for a few seconds to prevent any bleeding. Rub the site gently to close the needle track. Some bleeding may occur after the needle is pulled out; this is not harmful, although some insulin may be carried out with the blood. Press dry cotton firmly on the site. A clean finger also can be gently pressed over the site where the needle came out and rub the site gently. If an injection seems especially painful or if the blood or clear fluid is seen after withdrawing the needle, patient should apply firm pressure for 5 to 8 seconds at the site without rubbing. Blood glucose monitoring should be done more frequently on the day when this happens. If it is suspected that a significant portion of insulin dose was not administered, blood glucose should be checked within a few hours of the injection.

Pain can be minimized during injection by; injecting insulin at room temperature, removing all air bubbles before injection, waiting until topical alcohol has evaporated before injection, keeping muscles at the injection site relaxed while injecting, penetrating the skin quickly, not changing direction of the needle while inserting or withdrawing, not reusing needles. Prefilled syringes are stable for up to 30 days when kept in a refrigerator. If possible, the syringes should be stored with the needle pointing upward or lying flat, so that suspended insulin particles do not collect in the needle and clog it

Plugging of Needle

Occasionally, a small piece of fat or the insulin will plug the end of the needle during the injection. Sometimes it is possible to pull out the needle a little and then push the needle back into a slightly different place. If you still cannot push down the plunger to finish the injection, you have to use a new syringe. Note very precisely the units of insulin remaining in the plugged syringe. Fill a new syringe with the required insulin dose and inject into another site. Plugging of needles is not seen with insulin glargine and detemir.

Pen Devices for Insulin Injections

The introduction of the insulin pens was a milestone in insulin delivery. The first insulin pen, the NovoPen, was launched by Novo Nordisk in 1985. Because of increased convenience and portability, use of insulin pens has increased greatly in recent years. The required dose of insulin is dialed and the plunger is depressed after placing the needle in subcutaneous tissue.

Insulin pens can be disposable (use and throw the entire pen) or reusable (keep the pen permanently and replace the cartridges whenever necessary).

Pens for lispro, aspart, human NPH, premixed 30/70, Regular/NPH, glargine, detemir, premixed lispro, and premixed aspart are now widely available.

Some of the pen devices from **Novo-Nordisk** company that are available in the market include **NovoPen-4, NovoPen-5, FlexPen, FlexTouch and NovoPen-Echo. Out of these FlexTouch** is a disposable pen and NovoPen-Echo is especially convenient for children because ease of use. Some other brands of insulin pens are **HumaPen Ergo, Glaritus Pen Royale, INSUPen, and AllStar**.

Pen devices can deliver insulin from 0.5 to 70 units. The NovoPen-4 delivers a dose of 1 to 60 units. The BD pen has a maximum dose of 30 units.

Second-generation pen devices or "smart pens" with a memory function have been on the scene since 2007. The memory feature allows these devices to store the date, time, and amount of the previous doses. These devices are integrated with USB or Bluetooth features for efficient monitoring and data management. **HumaPen MEMOIR** is the world's first digital insulin pen with memory launched in 2007 by Eli Lilly followed by **HumaPen LUXURA HD**, a reusable pen for people who need insulin dosing in half-unit increments from 0.5 to 30 units. **NovoPen Echo**, the first insulin pen with memory and half-unit dosing features, was launched by Novo Nordisk in 2010. This device has several child-friendly attributes and displays time elapsed since the last dose.

Next generation insulin pens called connected pens (or smart pens use blue tooth and NFC (near field communication) to get connected to smart phones and other devices. **InPen System**, launched by Companion Medical, Novo Nordisk's **NovoPen 6 (Fig. 2.3) and NovoPen Echo Plus** fall into this category of pens. NovoPen 6 and NovoPen Echo Plus are reusable insulin pens equipped with NFC (near field communication) technology—meaning that they must be scanned in close proximity to move the data off the pen and to another device. The pens have an 800-injection dose memory and a remarkable five-year battery

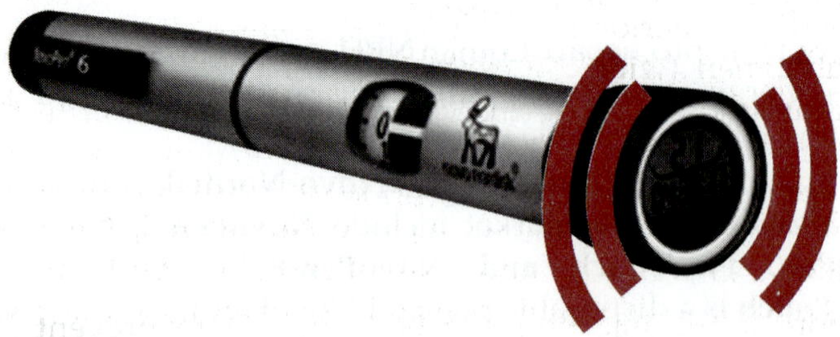

Fig. 2.3: NovoPen-6

life — no recharging is necessary, an advantage of using NFC. The NovoPen 6 and NovoPen Echo Plus both feature an electronic display that shows the amount of active insulin (insulin on board or "IOB"), size of the last dose and time since last injection.

Auto Injector Devices

Some people have difficulty pushing the needle through the skin. Also many people find it difficult to inject in areas difficult to reach such as the buttocks. Placing the syringe in an injection device such as the **Inject-Ease®**. After putting the syringe in the device and pushing a button, the needle is automatically pushed through the skin very quickly. It is still necessary to push down on the plunger of the syringe to inject the insulin.

Jet Injector Devices

Jet injector devices work by delivering a fine (0.008 inch) stream of insulin to the subcutaneous tissue under high pressure. They are virtually painless and are especially useful in children. The use of jet injections has been shown to alter the rate of absorption of subcutaneously injected insulin. Insulin is absorbed more rapidly after jet injection compare to syringe injection and the duration of action of intermediate acting insulins may be reduced which may be due to the availability of larger surface area for insulin absorption after dispersion of insulin dose by jet injection. **InsuJet** is one such device available in many countries.

Injection Sites

Insulin may be injected into the subcutaneous tissue of the upper arm and the anterior and lateral aspects of the thighs, buttocks and abdomen (with the exception of a circle with a 2-inch radius around the umbilicus. The abdomen has the fastest rate of absorption, followed by arms, thighs, and buttocks. Areas of lipohypertrophy slow the absorption **(Fig. 2.4)**.

Rotation of the Injection Sites

Rotation of the injection site is important to prevent lipo-hypertrophy or lipoatrophy. Rotating within one area is

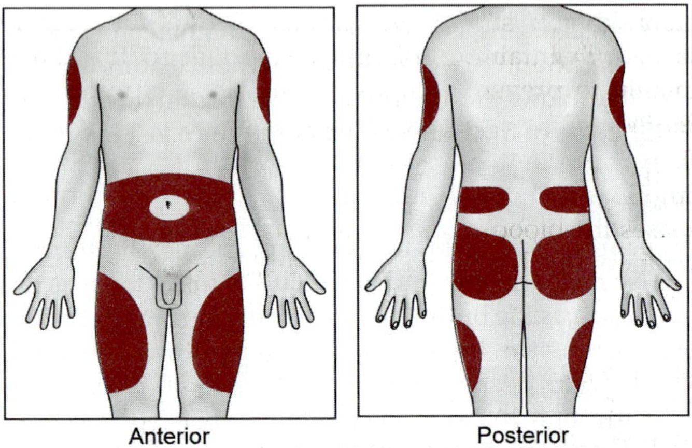

Fig. 2.4: Injection sites

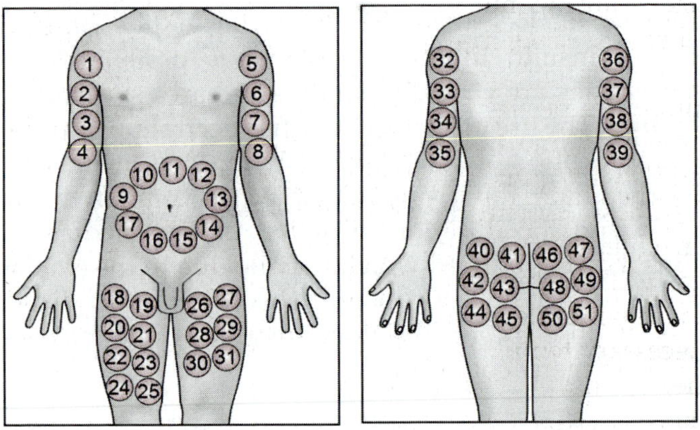

Fig. 2.5: Rotation of injection sites

recommended. For example, rotating injection systematically within the abdomen), rather than rotating to a different area with each injection.This will decrease variability of absorption from day to day **(Fig. 2.5)**.

Timing of Insulin Injections

Insulin lispro and aspart should be injected within 15 mins before a meal or with the meal or immediately after a meal.

Regular insulin should be injected 30 minutes before the meal. Not maintaining this much gap will reduce the ability of insulin to prevent a rapid rise in blood glucose and may increase the risk of delayed hypoglycemia.

It is important to avoid taking warm shower or bath or getting into a hot tub after taking insulin injection as this increases the blood supply to skin and results in faster rate of absorption which may result in hypoglycemia.

Injecting Insulin into Muscle

Intramuscular injections are not given routinely, and given only in special circumstances like DKA and HHS. It has faster rate of absorption than subcutaneous route.

In a person who is very thin or very muscular, there may be little fat under the skin. Injections may go into the underlying muscle, causing more rapid absorption of insulin and low blood sugar. There may then be less insulin to act later in the day, resulting in high blood sugar. Blood glucose should be monitored more frequently if it is suspected that insulin has been injected into the muscle. Injections into the muscle are most likely to occur if the syringe is held at a 90° angle to the body (unless short needles are used). Sometimes extra pain will occur when injections go into muscle, but this is not always the case. Thus, the pain is NOT a good indicator of injections given into muscle. If injecting into muscle is a problem, it may be necessary to pull the skin away from the muscle and insert the needle into the "tent" below while still holding the pinch of skin. Since the entire pinch is not being held, just the upper tip, the insulin should not leak-back. If the patient is newly diagnosed and has very little body fat, the buttocks may be the safest place for injections if he is injecting himself. With experience injecting into muscles will be rare.

Chapter

3

Different Types of Insulin Preparations

Two useful clinical classifications of insulin preparations are as follows.

Based on duration of Action

Rapid acting
Lispro, aspart, glulisine

Short acting
Regular insulin

Intermediate acting
NPH insulin (neutral protamine hagedorn, also called isophane insulin)

Long acting
Glargine, detemir, degludec

Based on Whether the Insulin Provides Prandial Coverage or Basal Coverage

Bolus or prandial insulins
Regular or plain insulin, lispro, aspart, glulisine

Basal insulins
NPH insulin, glargine, detemir, degludec

Regular and NPH insulins are also known as conventional (standard) preparations. They can be derived from beef, pork or recombinant-DNA technology (human insulin),

Lispro, aspart, glulisine, glargine, detemir and degludec are also called insulin analogues or designer insulins. They overcome some of the limitations of conventional insulin preparations. Insulin analogues are molecules that differ from human insulin in amino acid sequence but bind to same insulin receptors and function similarly as human insulin. Advantage of new insulin analogues is that they have better time–action profiles than conventional insulins.

Time–Action Profiles of Different Insulin Preparations after Subcutaneous Injection

Normal physiologic insulin secretion includes both a continuous basal (low-level) insulin secretion and an incremental postprandial secretion associated with meals. However, subcutaneously injected insulin takes sometime to get absorbed into blood stream and start its action. Following is the time–action profiles different insulin preparations after subcutaneous injection **(Fig. 3.1 and Table 3.1)**.

Table 3.1: Time–action profiles of different insulin preparations

Insulin formulation	*Onset of action*	*Peak action*	*Duration of action*
Lispro, Aspart, Glulisine	< 15 min	1 h	3–5 h
Regular (plain)	30 – 60 min	2–4 h	6–8 h
NPH	2–4 h	4–12 h	10–18 h
Glargine	2–4 h	No peak	24 h
Detemir	Slow	No peak	Up to 24 h
Degludec	1–2 h	No peak	Up to 42 h

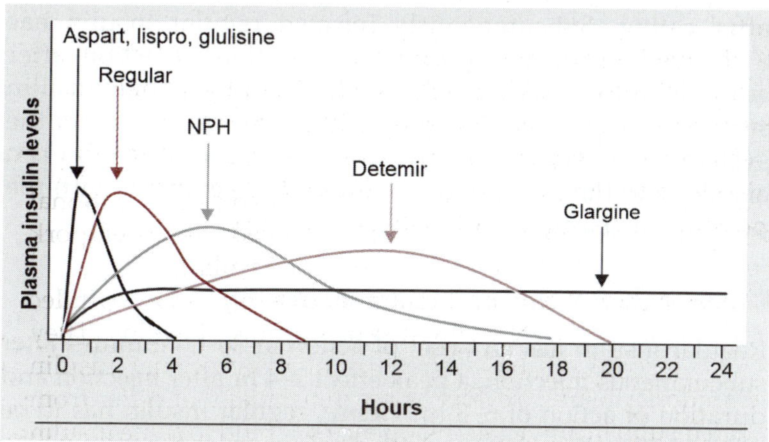

Fig. 3.1: Time–action profiles of different insulins

SHORT ACTING INSULINS

REGULAR INSULIN OR PLAIN INSULIN

Regular insulin has served the prototype of rapidly acting insulin for nearly the entire history of insulin therapy. It was earlier called rapid insulin. Now with the synthesis of newer insulin analogues which are rapid acting like insulin lispro and aspart, the term 'rapid acting' should not be used for regular insulin and instead should be used for lispro, aspart, and glulisine.

In nondiabetic person serum level of insulin rises rapidly after meal ingestion from basal levels of 5–20 μU/ml to peak levels of 80–120 μU/ml in 30–60 minutes after a high carbohydrate meal. Insulin secreted from pancreas enters portal circulation first and hence portal insulin concentrations are 2–3 fold higher than systemic insulin levels as the blood has to pass through liver first. This high concentration of insulin inhibits hepatic glucose output and hence helps in maintaining euglycemia. Because of all these, a non-diabetic person shows only a mild increase in blood glucose level after a meal.

Subcutaneously injected regular insulin cannot mimic the physiologic pattern of endogenous insulin secretion after eating. Subcutaneously injected regular insulin has a delayed onset and prolonged duration of action after administration making reproduction of physiologic insulin secretion impossible. Exogenously given insulin enters the systemic circulation directly. Long-term use of insulin can also lead to the production of antibodies against it with the possible development of insulin resistance.

Time–Action Profile of Regular Insulin (Fig. 3.1)

Regular insulin has an onset of action in 30–60 minutes after subcutaneous injection, a peak effect 2–4 hr after injection and duration of action of 6–8 hr. Hence, regular insulin has to be injected 30 to 40 minutes before meals in order to optimize the postprandial hyperglycemia.

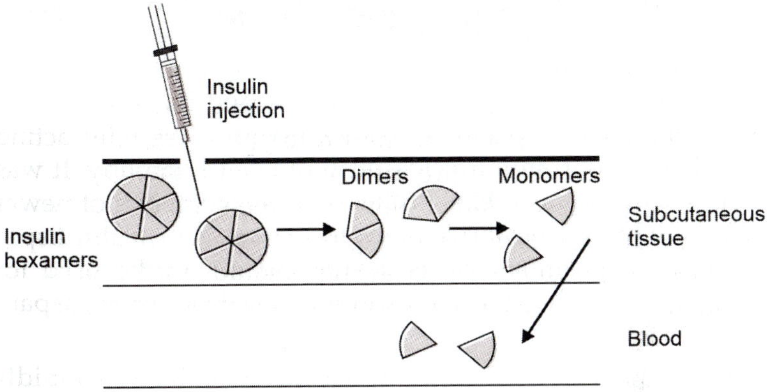

Fig. 3.2: Regular insulin absorption after subcutaneous injection

Insulin molecules are stored as hexamer form in beta cells of pancreas. The formation of hexamers is due to the presence of zinc. When secreted from the beta cells, the zinc gets released and hexamers dissociate into monomers which is the active form of insulin. Same thing happens with regular insulin preparation. Zinc is added to regular insulin and there is formation of insulin hexamers. When insulin is injected into subcutaneous tissue, zinc is released due to dilution, and insulin hexamers dissociate into dimers and then into monomers **(Fig. 3.2)**. Monomers are then absorbed into blood stream. This dissociation of insulin hexamers into monomers takes sometime leading to delayed onset of action of regular insulin.

INSULIN LISPRO

Insulin lispro was introduced in 1996. Lispro insulin is produced by interchanging two amino acids on beta chain, i.e. proline at B-28, and lysine at B-29. The first three letters of lysine and proline were combined to name it as Lyspro. Subsequently Lyspro was changed to Lispro since it was planned to release this all over the world and as some languages donot contain the letter "Y". Lispro insulin is at least twice as fast acting as regular human insulin.

In contrast to regular insulin where insulin monomers aggregate to form hexamers, lispro insulin molecules do not aggregate to form hexamers and remain in monomeric form. Hence, lispro insulin gets absorbed fast and has rapid onset of action. This property of insulin lispro is because of the interchange of 2 amino acids on β-chain, i.e. proline at B28 position and lysine at B29. Proline residue in the 28th position of β-chain has a crucial role in the formation of insulin dimers. Changing its position reduces the formation of dimers without changing the biological activity of the molecule.

Time–Action Profile of Insulin Lispro (Fig. 3.1)

After SC administration lispro begins acting within 15 mins, reaches peak concentrations between 30 and 60 minutes, peaks in activity in 60 to 90 minutes and has a duration of action of 3–5 hr. Peak insulin action occurs approximately twice as fast with the lispro as with regular insulin. Because of its fast onset of action, lispro can be given within 15 minutes before meals. It can also be given immediately before or after meals. After taking injection, there is no need to wait for 30 mins to take meals like regular insulin, hence lispro is also called no wait insulin.

The formation of antibodies to lispro is similar to that of human insulin. These antibodies usually decrease over time.

Advantages of Insulin Lispro Over Regular (Plain) Insulin

- Lispro is as effective as regular (plain) insulin and its peak concentrations are 2–3 times higher than regular insulin. It has better ability to mimic physiological pattern of insulin secretion than regular insulin. Because of its more rapid onset and peak action, insulin lispro more effectively controls postprandial blood sugar at 1 and 2 hr than regular insulin.
- Lispro is more effective in suppressing hepatic glucose output than regular insulin, because of higher concentrations attained in liver.
- The onset of action of lispro does not vary much with the site of injection as compared to regular insulin but when injected

into deltoid or thigh, lispro exhibits a slightly prolonged duration of action.

- Lispro has less intra-individual and inter-individual variations compared to regular insulin due to predictable absorption. Regular insulin has to be injected 30–40 minutes before a meal, whereas lispro can be injected 0–15 minutes before a meal and this achieves postprandial glycemic control that is as good as or better than regular insulin. This applies to both pump administration and subcutaneous injection.
- The more rapid peak and shorter duration of action of lispro makes late postprandial hypoglycemia less of a problem than with regular insulin. This advantage is especially apparent at night in patients with tight glucose control. A large meta-analysis that represented more than 1400 patient-years reported a 25 percent reduction in the frequency of severe hypoglycemia (i.e., that which required the assistance of another person to correct) with the use of insulin lispro, as compared with regular insulin.
- A potential advantage of insulin lispro is in children, who are fussy eaters. Many parents worry when they give regular insulin to a child before meal and then the child does not eat adequate food or decides not to eat. This may cause hypoglycemia in the child. However, this potential cause for worry may be avoided with lispro insulin as it can be given after the child has finished eating without significantly compromising the postprandial blood sugar control.
- Lispro can also be adjusted according to the meal size any time during the day or night. The increase in dose of regular insulin to cover a huge dinner may cause nocturnal hypoglycemia which is not seen with insulin lispro. This flexibility of lispro would be welcomed by many patients.
- Use of insulin lispro also simplifies exercise programme in diabetics. With regular insulin use, unanticipated exercise 3–4 hr after the injection may result in hypoglycemia unless adequate carbohydrate is consumed to avoid it. This is not so with lispro insulin because its action does not last so long as it gets over by 2 – 2 ½ hr after the injection. However, exercising 5 hr after insulin lispro injection may increase blood sugar

levels. This happens because after 5 hr there won't be insulin lispro in the blood and in the absence of insulin, exercise induces glucose raising counter regulatory responses.

- Lispro can be used interchangeably with other insulins. Lispro can be used at one meal and regular insulin at other meal.

Though there were controversies about the increased incidence of late postprandial hyperglycemia with lispro compared to regular insulin, a recent study has demonstrated that early waning of the lispro activity does not result in postprandial hyperglycemia and the reduction in blood glucose effected by lispro is consistent and stable for 8 hr after meal ingestion if adequate doses are used.

Pregnant Women

Data from prospective, blinded, randomized clinical trials of insulin analogues in pregnancy are lacking. However, retrospective studies have not shown any significant difference between insulin lispro and regular insulin with regard to either fetal or maternal outcomes. Maximum data regarding safety in pregnancy for any insulin analogue is for insulin lispro. Most experts now agree that insulin lispro can be used safely in pregnancy.

Summarizing insulin lispro, though insulin lispro has got many advantages over regular insulin, clinical trials have shown that it does not appear to alter overall control (as measured by hemoglobin A1C levels) and at present there is no indication for replacing regular insulin with insulin lispro in the majority of patients. However, it may help patients whose mealtimes are unpredictable, those with poor postprandial sugar control, and those who eat late in the evening and are prone to early nocturnal hypoglycemia.

Note: Do not use lispro with alpha glucosidase inhibitors (acarbose, voglibose) as these drugs delay the absorption of glucose. This may cause hypoglycemia as lispro acts fast.

INSULIN ASPART

The second rapidly acting analogue that was introduced is insulin aspart. It was released in 2001. In insulin aspart, neutral proline in B-28 position is replaced by the negatively charged aspartic acid resulting in reduced capacity for self-association and faster absorption.

Time–Action Profile of Aspart

The time–action profile of aspart is similar to insulin lispro. Because of its fast action profile, it can be administered immediately before meals. It can be administered after meals also.

Clinical Efficacy

Many clinical trials have shown that insulin aspart is as effective as human insulin in diabetic patients. Insulin aspart is superior to regular insulin in the reduction of postprandial hyperglycemia. Except in the case of insulin-pump therapy, insulin aspart is used only as prandial insulin replacement. In insulin pump therapy, it provides both basal and prandial insulin. In general, studies involving multiple daily injections have not demonstrated that rapidly acting analogues improve glycosylated hemoglobin levels better than conventional insulins. Nevertheless, it appears that an improvement in the control of postprandial hyperglycemia, which is not well captured by glycosylated hemoglobin, may be important in preventing or delaying diabetes-related complications. Due to better control of postprandial hyperglycemia, rapidly acting analogues (particularly in combination with long-acting analogues or continuous subcutaneous infusion of insulin) could have a greater effect than regular insulin on the reduction of complications of diabetes. In addition, studies have shown that rapidly acting analogues are superior to regular insulin for lowering glycosylated hemoglobin levels in patients who receive insulin by continuous subcutaneous infusion.

Insulin Aspart in Pregnant Women

Treatment with insulin aspart was associated with a tendency toward fewer fetal losses and preterm deliveries than treatment with human insulin. Insulin aspart could not be detected in the fetal circulation and no increase in insulin antibodies was found. Thus, the use of insulin aspart in pregnancy is regarded safe.

FAST ACTING INSULIN ASPART

Fast acting insulin aspart (faster aspart) is insulin aspart with two added excipients, L-arginine and niacinamide, to ensure formulation stability with accelerated initial absorption after subcutaneous administration compared with normal aspart.

Clinical trials have shown that faster aspart has even more faster onset of action compared to normal aspart, and achieves higher concentration in the blood after meal thus providing superior postprandial blood glucose control. Its action gets over much earlier than normal aspart thus reducing the chances of hypoglycemia before the next meal. Because of all these advantages faster aspart more closely mimics the physiological action of insulin secreted by the pancreas with improved glycemic control.

In addition, faster aspart administered up to 20 min after the start of a meal was noninferior to mealtime normal aspart in terms of A1C control, highlighting the opportunity for postmeal injection.

INSULIN GLULISINE

Insulin glulisine is a new rapidly acting analogue with a pharmacokinetic profile that is similar to those of insulin lispro and insulin aspart. Glulisine differs from regular insulin by the replacement of asparagine by lysine at position B3 and lysine by glutamic acid at B29. These modifications in glulisine allow it to exist as more stable dimers and monomers, allowing glulisine to be suspended in a zinc-free buffer, unlike regular insulin and other rapid-acting insulin analogues like lispro and aspart.

Studies have shown that glulisine has more rapid onset of action than lispro and aspart and also attains more serum concentration after subcutaneous injection than lispro which makes it more useful to control postprandial hyperglycemia.

Glulisine can be used as subcutaneous injection, continuous subcutaneous infusion and also intravenously.

Glulisine can be used in children older than 4 years of age. Available data suggest that there are no adverse effects on fetus if used during pregnancy and also no adverse effect on infant if used during lactation.

Glulisine can be used in patients with renal and hepatic impairment but should be monitored carefully for hypoglycemia.

INTERMEDIATE ACTING INSULINS

NPH INSULIN AND LENTE INSULINS

NPH (neutral protamine hagedorn) insulin is produced by complexing regular insulin with protamine, a protein of fish origin and adding trace amounts of zinc. The protamine insulin complex is poorly soluble at physiologic pH and thus slowly absorbed from the subcutaneous tissue. Hagedorn is the name of the scientist who first formulated this preparation.

Lente insulin is no longer being used in human beings, but still being used in veterinary practice.

NPH is labeled as "N" on bottles. NPH insulin is now being produced by DNA recombinant technology.

Time Action Profile NPH Insulin (Fig. 3.1)

NPH insulin has an onset of action within 2 – 4 hours of injection, a peak action 4–12 hours after injection, and a duration of action of 10–18 hours.

NPH insulin has a somewhat higher risk of hypoglycemia. Inadequate resuspension is thought to contribute to the high day-to-day variability in the pharmacodynamic and pharmacokinetic profile of NPH insulin, leading to hypoglycemia. Patients can adequately resuspend NPH by rotating the vial several times until it is uniformly cloudy. Nocturnal hypoglycemia is another risk when NPH is given in the night. With night dose, NPH peak occurs at midnight when the body does not require as much insulin and this may cause nocturnal hypoglycemia.

NPH can be mixed with regular insulin and such premixed preparations are available in the market (e.g. Mixtard 70/30 where 70% is NPH insulin and 30% is human regular insulin). NPH is not an ideal basal insulin because its action does not last throughout the day and it has a peak action. Ideal basal insulin works throughout the day and provides constant basal level without any peak. *NPH insulin should not be given intravenously.*

Other intermediate acting insulins are insulin aspart protamine and insulin lispro protamine. Here the rapid acting aspart and lispro are made intermediate acting by adding protamine.

LONG ACTING INSULINS

INSULIN GLARGINE

Insulin glargine is a long acting human insulin analogue produced by recombinant- DNA technology. It was introduced in 2001. This is the first true basal insulin. The structure of insulin glargine differs from that of human insulin in that glycine replaces asparagine at position 21 of the A-chain, and two arginines are added to the C-terminus of the B-chain. These changes give unique properties to insulin glargine which remains completely soluble in the acidic pH of the vial (pH 4) but precipitates in the neutral pH of subcutaneous tissue after injection. Insulin glargine is then slowly released from these precipitates, producing a relatively constant plasma insulin levels over 24 hr with no pronounced peaks. This allows once a day subcutaneous injection of insulin, which can provide basal levels of insulin throughout the day.

The commercially available formulation of insulin glargine also contains a small amount of zinc (30 ug/ml), which facilitates the formation of micro precipitates in the neutral pH of subcutaneous tissue. At clinically relevant concentrations, insulin receptor binding is similar to regular insulin. Insulin glargine is well tolerated and is not associated with greater immunogenicity or weight gain than NPH insulin. It is also suitable as initial insulin therapy in both type 1 and type 2 diabetes. It is safe for use in children and adolescents. However, data are not available about its use in pregnant women.

Time–Action Profile of Insulin Glargine

As compared with NPH insulin, insulin glargine results in prolonged insulin absorption and shows little peak activity. Rates of absorption of insulin glargine at various sites do not differ and it does not accumulate after multiple injections. It has its onset of action in 2–4 hours. Its activity in normal volunteers lasts for up to 30 hours. In another pharmacodynamic study, insulin glargine was found to have no peak and to have a mean duration of action of 22 ± 4 hours. Steady plasma concentrations of insulin are achieved 2 to 4 days after the first dose and no accumulation of insulin glargine occurs after repeated daily doses. There is partial degradation of insulin glargine in subcutaneous tissues into two active products. Hence, both unchanged drug and metabolites are present in the blood. There may be some inter and intra individual variation in the time–action profile of insulin glargine.

Advantages

- Many trials have shown better control of fasting blood glucose levels and decreased incidence of nocturnal hypoglycemia compared to NPH insulin in both type 1 and type 2 DM.
- There is also more improvement in HbA1C levels than with NPH insulin.
- The site of injection does not alter the time action profile of insulin glargine.
- The time of the day at which insulin glargine is injected does not alter glycemic control.
- The plasma levels of insulin glargine do not fluctuate significantly, thus mimicking physiological basal insulin profile.

Interactions with other Drugs

Blood glucose lowering effect of insulin glargine is potentiated by oral antidiabetic agents, ACE inhibitors, dextropropoxyphene, disopyramide, fibrates, fluoxetine, MAO inhibitors, pentoxifylline, salicylates and sulfonamide antibacterials

Blood glucose lowering effect of insulin glargine is attenuated by corticosteroids, danazol, progesterones, phenothiazine derivatives, somatropin, sympathomimetics (adrenaline, salbutamol) and thyroid hormones.

Others that may affect the glucose lowering effect of insulin glargine are beta blockers, clonidine, lithium, and alcohol.

Glargine solution is clear and slightly acidic (pH 4) and should not be mixed with any other insulin or solution as this could alter its time–action profile.

Tolerability

Incidence of adverse events is similar to that seen with NPH insulin. Injection site reactions are the most common type of adverse events and are seen in 3 to 4% of patients. These reactions include redness, pain, itching, hives, swelling, or inflammation at the site of injection. Most of these reactions are minor, do not require discontinuation of therapy, and resolve within a few days or weeks. Lipodystrophy, which may be seen with any type of insulin therapy can be minimized or prevented by rotation of injection sites. Antibody formation against insulin glargine is no greater than NPH insulin and is clinically insignificant

Pregnancy

Insulin glargine is considered safe during pregnancy, and there are no known risks of infant harm if using the medication during lactation. However, the FDA lists insulin glargine as category C in pregnancy, stating that the patient should only use it if the benefits outweigh the risk.

Children

FDA has approved use of glargine in children of 6 years and above. However, studies have shown the safety of glargine in children below 6 years of age also.

Renal and Liver Impairment

In both renal and liver disease patients, blood glucose should be monitored frequently and dose adjusted accordingly to prevent hypoglycemia.

Place of Insulin Glargine in the Management of Diabetes

It is indicated for the treatment of adults or children (aged >6 yr) with type 1 diabetes and adults with type 2 diabetes. It provides basal insulin levels and is given as once daily subcutaneous injection. Numerous clinical trials have documented that insulin glargine is more effective in glycemic control than NPH insulin as evidenced by improved HbA1c levels. It is associated with decreased frequency of nocturnal hypoglycemia attacks compared to NPH insulin. These findings apply both to type 1 and type 2 DM. Weight gain is no more than with NPH insulin.

In normal people there is continuous secretion of insulin known as basal insulin secretion with increased secretion following meals. These postprandial peaks of insulin can be mimicked by giving short acting insulin (regular or lispro) before or with the meals. However, the problem was with regard to replacing basal insulin secretion. This would require insulin which acts throughout the day without any peak. Though NPH partially satisfies this requirement, it has a peak effect, which may produce hypoglycemia. When this peak corresponds to postprandial hyperglycemia, it controls blood sugar, but when the peak occurs at other times, it may produce hypoglycemia. Another disadvantage of NPH is unpredictable absorption from the injection site. Insulin glargine satisfies most requirements of a basal insulin because of its peakless, prolonged duration of action and predictable absorption from any subcutaneous injection site. Hence, the discovery of insulin glargine has been a great step ahead in the control of diabetes.

Based on evidence of efficacy in the form of glycemic control and potential avoidance of hypoglycemic episodes, insulin glargine is recommended as a treatment option in both type 1 and type 2 DM. However, if the glycemic control and HbA1c are good with other insulin preparations and there is no frequent hypoglycemia, a change to glargine is probably not needed. ("if it is not broken, donot fix it."!). Similarly, if the patient is not ready for three or four injections per day, glargine should not be considered.

Disadvantages of Insulin Glargine

- No other insulin can be mixed in the same syringe. It is more acidic (pH 4.0) than other insulins (pH 7.4). If insulin glargine is mixed with another insulin, time action profile of both insulins change.
- When using insulin glargine,three or more injections per day of a short-acting insulin may be needed before meals.
- Because the solution is clear, care must be taken not to confuse it with the short-acting insulin.

INSULIN DETEMIR

Detemir, another new long-acting insulin analogue is acylated analogue of human insulin. Here, the amino acid threonine at the B-30 position on the human insulin chain is lacking and a 14-carbon fatty acid (tetradecanoic acid or myristic acid) is attached to lysine at B-29. It is a clear solution and remains as a solution after subcutaneous injection without precipitation. It is a soluble basal insulin analogue with a neutral pH. It has a high affinity for serum albumin from which it gets released slowly which accounts for its unique mechanism of prolonged duration of action. The shelf life of detemir is 2 years but after opening the product, it can be stored for a maximum of 6 weeks.

Time–Action Profile of Insulin Detemir

Insulin detemir has a flat action profile than NPH insulin. Its duration of action depends on the dose injected also. At doses of 0.1– 0.2 units/kg body wt, detemir has flat action profile and acts nearly for 24 hours. Higher doses than this cause slight peaking of insulin action and prolong the duration of action to more than 24 hours.

Some reports suggest that it has duration of action of only 20 hr, which means that it may have to be given twice daily to provide round the clock basal insulin coverage. When given twice daily steady state serum concentrations are reached after 2–3 injections.

Advantages of Insulin Detemir

Absorption and action of insulin detemir is more predictable because of two reasons. Since detemir is a clear solution, it does not require resuspension. Another reason is detemir remains liquid after subcutaneous injection and does not precipitate. This also accounts for uniform predictable action since a precipitated depot leads to unpredictable absorption. Detemir also has prominent action on hepatic glucose output which may be an advantage not seen with other insulins.

Safety of Insulin Detemir

Detemir pharmacokinetics is similar in children, adolescents, and adults. The IGF receptor affinity of detemir is less than human insulin; hence, there is no risk of carcinogenicity. No drug interactions between insulin detemir and other albumin bound drugs have been observed *in vitro* studies. Neither renal nor hepatic impairment exert clinically important influences on the pharmacokinetic profile of insulin detemir. No adequate data are available for its use during pregnancy and it should be avoided in pregnancy. Detemir should not be mixed with any IV fluids.

Summary of Insulin Detemir

- Insulin detemir is a basal insulin analogue.
- Insulin detemir acts for up to 24 hours. It can be administered once or twice daily depending on the patients needs in combination with meal related short or rapid acting insulin.
- Insulin detemir appears to provide more stable glycaemic control with less risk of nocturnal hypoglycemia.
- Weight gain is less with detemir than NPH. In clinical trials, patients using NPH insulin gained an average 0.6 kg more weight than those on insulin detemir.

INSULIN DEGLUDEC

This is a new ultra-long acting insulin analogue. Insulin degludec (available with the brand name Tresiba) differs from human insulin in that the amino acid threonine in position B30 has been omitted and a side-chain consisting of glutamic acid and a C16 fatty acid has been attached. These changes allow for the formation of multi-hexamers. When injected subcutaneously, these multi-hexamers form a drug depot store from which monomers are slowly and continuously released accounting for prolonged duration of action of up to 42 hours. Compared to other long acting basal insulins such as glargine and detemir, which have a duration of action of 20–24 hours, insulin degludec provides a consistent level of basal insulin over 42 hours with a low peak:trough ratio. Degludec has low intra-individual variability and plasma concentration is less dependent on the time of injections. Thus it has flexibility in dose timing and predicatbale long duration of action with low risk of hypoglycemia.

Degludec is a clear, colorless solution with a pH-dependent solubility and an isoelectric point similar to that of human insulin, and it is administered subcutaneously.

Compared with glargine, degludec is associated with equivalent HbA1c control and significantly lower nocturnal hypoglycemia rates. Degludec is also associated with significantly greater reductions in FPG and lower total doses of insulin versus glargine

Degludec can be used in children aged 1 year and above. Degludec is not recommended during pregnancy due to lack of safety studies. However, some studies have shown no fetal side-effects. Hence if clinically indicated, it can be considered during pregnancy. There is no clinical experience with degludec during breastfeeding. It is unknown whether it is excreted into breast milk.

Degludec can also be used in renal and hepatic impairment.

A premixed combination of degludec (70%) and aspart (30%) is now available. It is called IDegAsp. This is the first basal bolus insulin premix. The advantage of this IDegAsp premix insulin is that it reduces the number of insulin injections compared to basal bolus regimen. We know that in basal bolus regimen, we have to inject short acting insulin before every meal (i.e. three times) and one injection of basal insulin daily.

This makes four injections per day which reduces compliance as patients are reluctant to take four injections per day. With IDegAsp the number of injections can be reduced to three as this premix can be given before breakfast (one injection which takes care of basal requirement as well as prandial requirement after breakfast) and aspart alone is given before lunch and dinner to take care of prandial requirement (two injections). Studies have shown that even two injections of IDegAsp (one injection before breakfast and one before dinner) is effective in achieving glycemic control with less risk of hypoglycemia.

Summarizing the available data on insulin degludec, it has many advantages over other basal insulins such as glargine and detemir. Degludec has the flexibility of taking it at any time of the day, with an acceptable interinjection period of 8–42 hours, and less chances of hypoglycemia. Another advantage is that it can be mixed with short acting insulins such as aspart to reduce the number of injections taken per day.

BASAL INSULIN Fc (BIF) AND INSULIN ICODEC (once a week insulins)

These two insulins are even more long acting than insulin degludec. Both these insulins can be given once weekly. This will reduce the number of injections in basal bolus regimen since any of the above basal insulins can be given once weekly. In addition, type 2 diabetics who are initiated on once daily basal insulin can be given once a week injection if the trials on above two insulins become successful.

So far, in phase 2 trials Basal Insulin Fc (BIF) has been shown to be similar to degludec in reducing A1C, with a similar risk of hypoglycemia.

Insulin Icodec is in phase 3 trials. So far studies have shown that insulin icodec has almost similar effect to that of degludec in terms of reducing HbA1C in both type 1 and type 2 diabetes. Insulin icodec was superior to glargine in people with type 2 DM. Rates of severe hypoglycemia were statistically the same between icodec and glargine in people with type 2 DM. Rates of severe hypoglycemia were significantly higher in the icodec group than in the degludec group in people with type 1 DM.

Chapter

4

Initiation of Insulin in Diabetes

Starting insulin can be sometimes difficult because patients often have misconceptions about insulin. Many have fear of injections and worry about decreased flexibility of lifestyle. Patients often have a fear of the injection being painful or not being able to inject them. These fears should be addressed by discussion and demonstrating how painless the injection actually is. An insulin injection device will solve many of these problems and is suitable for most patients. In some states, getting driving license may be difficult for those who are on insulin. All available alternatives should be tried for such patients before deciding on insulin use. Those who have problems with injection due to visual impairment, poor manual dexterity and/or cognitive impairment, insulin can be administered by a relative, caregiver or a nurse if necessary.

Once it is decided that a patient requires insulin, the need for insulin injections and its benefit should be explained to the patient. Patients should not be made to feel that it is because of their failure that the insulin is being considered, even if noncompliance with diet and exercise has contributed to this. Patients require education about insulin injection skills and the need for monitoring blood sugar regularly. Patients should also be educated about recognizing hypoglycemia and corrective steps to prevent and treat it. Eating patterns may need to be adjusted including introduction of snacks in between meals. Weight gain is common with insulin therapy and every effort should be made to prevent or minimize it through dietary regulation and physical activity.

INITIATION OF INSULIN IN TYPE 1 DIABETES

Insulin replacement is necessary for all patients with type 1 DM from the time of diagnosis and involves multiple daily injections. Type 1 DM patients present usually with the classical symptoms of polyphagia, polydypsia, and polyuria. They may also present with complications like infections, DKA and HHS etc, and this may be the first time that they are detected to have DM. If the patient presents with any of these complications admit the patient and start insulin. If no complications, insulin can be started on OPD basis provided patient monitors his blood glucose and comes for frequent review or maintains telephone contact with doctor.

Insulin requirements are difficult to predict in newly diagnosed patients and may change rapidly because lowering blood glucose and the alleviation of glucotoxicity on the beta-cell will allow endogenous insulin secretory reserve to recover. In some patients this may lead to a prolonged 'honeymoon', period, sometimes lasting months, during which insulin requirements fall dramatically. During this period, good glucose control can be maintained with little or no exogenous insulin.

How to Choose the Initial Total Dose of Insulin for Type 1 DM Patients

The insulin dose required for a type I diabetic patient, within 20% of their ideal body wt in the absence of intercurrent infection or other periods of instability, ***approximates 0.4 to 1 unit/kg/day***. During periods of relative remission ("honeymoon period") during which beta-cell activity may increase, requirements may be less. During periods of intercurrent illness, insulin requirements may be high. Requirement is also high during adolescent growth spurt. It is always safer to initiate insulin at the dose of 0.4 units/kg/day to avoid hypoglycemia. Higher doses such as 0.7 units/kg/day may be used in the presence of ketone bodies. Once the total dose is calculated based on body weight, approximately half (40 to 60%) of the total dose is given as basal insulin and remaining half (40 to 60%) is given as prandial insulin.

Suppose a type-1 diabetic patient weighs 60 kg, now his total insulin requirement per day is 0.4 units multiplied by 60, i,e. 24 units per day. Half of this 24 units, i.e. 12 units is given as basal insulin and remaining half (i.e. 12 units) is given as prandial insulin. This 12 units of prandial insulin is further divided and given as 4 units before the three major meals (4 units before breakfast, 4 units before lunch, and 4 units before dinner). Remember that these initial doses have to be adjusted based on blood sugar measurements once in 2 to 3 days.

Options for basal insulin are NPH, glargine, detemir, and degludec. We can choose any basal insulin, but it is better to choose one of the latest long acting basal insulins such as glargine or detemir or degludec rather than NPH, because these latest basal insulins act throughout the day with reduced risk of hypoglycemia as compared to NPH which has to be given twice daily and has higher chances of hypoglycemia.

Options for prandial insulin (given before every meal) are regular insulin, lispro, aspart, fast acting aspart, and glulisine. Lispro, aspart, and glulisine have less chances of causing postprandial hypoglycemia and also more effectively control postprandial surge of blood glucose. Hence, these are preferred over human insulin.

Type 1 diabetes patients usually require multiple insulin injection regimens to achieve blood sugar control. Some patients may achieve adequate sugar control with twice-daily injection of short-acting plus intermediate acting insulin (using premixed preparations or manually mixed before injection). However, most type 1 diabetics require three or more injections using basal bolus therapy.

If using premixed preparation, two-thirds of the total required dose is given before breakfast, and remaining one-third should be given in the night before dinner. Injection should be given 30 minutes before meals if using premixed human insulin preparation (regular plus NPH premixed in the ratio of 30:70).

Summary of Initiation of Insulin in Type 1 Diabetes **(Table 4.1)**

Table 4.1: Total initial dose per day = 0.4 to 0.1 units per kg body weight ·

Basal bolus regimen (one injection of basal insulin and three injections of prandial insulin before every meal)	
Basal insulin 1st choice: Glargine or degludec once daily 2nd choice: Detemir once daily 3rd choice: NPH twice daily	Total insulin dose required per day is divided as basal 40–60% and prandial 40–60%. Prandial insulin is equally divided and given before every meal If using glargine or detemir as basal insulin it should not be mixed with any short-acting insulin because of physicochemical incompatibility. Glargine or detemir is given at bedtime once daily. Short-acting insulin such as lispro or aspart are given before every meal. This works out to 4 injections per day (1 basal and 3 mealtime injections)
Prandial insulin (three times per day, i.e. before every meal) 1st choice: Lispro or aspart or glulisine 2nd choice: Faster acting aspart 3rd choice: Regular human insulin	If using degludec as basal injection either it can be injected separately at any time of the day or it can be mixed with short-acting insulin. Premixed preparation of degludec and aspart is available in the ratio of 30:70, which can be injected before a major meal. This brings down the number of injections to 3 per day instead of 4
Continuous subcutaneous insulin infusion (CSII)	
Any short-acting insulin can be used 1st choice: Lispro or aspart 2nd choice: Faster acting aspart 3rd choice: Regular human insulin	40–50% of the total dose is given as basal dose, i.e. as continuous infusion over 24 hours. Remaining insulin is divided equally and given 15 to 20 minutes before every meal
Twice or thrice daily premixed insulin (not ideal for type-1 diabetes)	
Mix of regular insulin and NPH (30:70 or 50:50 ratio)	This is given twice daily (before breakfast and dinner). However, this is not the ideal regimen in type 1 diabetics but may work in some patients

Contd...

Contd...

Twice or thrice daily premixed insulin (not ideal for type-1 diabetes)	
Mix of aspart and protamine aspart (25:75 or 50:50 ratio)	This is given two times per day (one injection before breakfast and another before dinner) OR Thrice daily (one injection before every meal)
Mix of lispro and insulin lispro protamine (25:75 or 50:50 ratio)	This is given two times per day (one injection before breakfast and another before dinner) OR Thrice daily (one injection before every meal)

For further details, see Chapter 5 on insulin injection regimens.

INITIATION OF INSULIN IN TYPE 2 DIABETES

Type 2 diabetes is well recognized as a chronic and progressive disease. Insulin resistance is the main problem here. The initial response to insulin resistance is increased secretion of insulin from beta cells of pancreas. This increased secretion of insulin reaches a peak at some point of time and then gradually starts declining as a result of gradual decline in beta cell function. Thereafter the natural history of the disease is such that beta cell function continues to deteriorate and glycemic control gets more and more difficult.

Lifestyle changes and certain oral antidiabetic agents such as metformin and thiazolidinediones, can improve insulin sensitivity and in theory slow decline of beta cell function. However, in practice, the former is very difficult to achieve and the latter seems to exert only a modest effect. Another unfortunate thing is that type 2 diabetes is affecting more and more young people including teenagers. As a result, the number of patients reaching the point of failure on maximum tolerated doses of oral antidiabetic drugs is increasing very fast.

As the disease progresses and beta cell function declines, most people will require insulin. In an evaluation of more than 2700 UKPDS patients followed for 6 yr, 30% of those taking sulphonylureas and 22% of those taking metformin required insulin therapy because they became symptomatic or developed fasting glucose levels of $\geq$ 270 mg/dL within 6 yr of follow up. Most patients will require insulin over the course of 15 yr or so.

Indications for Insulin Treatment in Type 2 Diabetes

Absolute Indications

1. Diabetic ketaocidosis or HHS
2. Presence of serious infection or concurrent illness (e.g. acute M1, pancreatitis or stroke).
3. Surgery
4. Pregnancy; all pregnant women with diabetes mellitus, (whether gestational or previous diabetes) whose disease is not controlled with diet alone should be treated with insulin. All oral agents are contraindicated during pregnancy except metformin, which is relatively safe.

Relative Indications

1. Symptomatic (polydypsia, polyuria, polyphagia and wt loss) uncontrolled diabetes, with persistent elevations of the FBS levels of 300 mg/dL or higher. Intensive insulin therapy with tight glycemic control helps reverse glucose toxicity. Therapy improves both insulin sensitivity and insulin secretion. After 6–8 wk of good glycemic control, these patients can be switched to an oral agent or can continue insulin therapy.
2. Onset prior to age 30, as they may not respond adequately to oral agents.
3. Wt loss or below ideal body weight, as insulin therapy will normalize metabolic derangements and helps in weight gain.
4. High dose glucocorticoids causing hyperglycemia, as this will not respond to oral agents.

Some of the above indications are temporary, e.g. all the absolute indications listed above are temporary indications, and oral agents may be restarted once the indication is over. However, some patients may require permanent conversion to insulin.

Who should be considered for conversion to insulin on permanent basis?

1. Failure to achieve recommended targets with 3 or more oral agents.

2. Over 15 yr duration of diabetes, as by this time there may be complete loss of β-cell function
3. Patients who after discussing the treatment options with physician, wishes to receive insulin as initial therapy

Alternatives to Insulin

Before starting insulin for type 2 diabetic patients, try the following if feasible:

- Many patients fail on oral antidiabetic drugs because of poor compliance with drugs, diet, and exercise. Any one or all of these may be responsible. Compliance may be improved dramatically by the mere mention of insulin injections, as many will worry about having to take injections. Dietary compliance should be checked and reinforced. Compliance with drugs may also be improved by changing a twice-daily sulphonylurea to one of the newer once-daily preparations such as glimepiride or Glipizide-SR, or long acting preparation of metformin.
- Thiozolidinediones (TZD), alpha glucosidase inhibitors (Acarbose, Voglibose), and SGLT2 inhibitors (canagliflozin, dapagliflozin, and empagliflozin) may be added if the patient is not already on these drugs. Sometimes addition of these drugs may bring the sugar under control even without insulin.

Insulin Initiation Strategies in Type 2 Diabetes

Choosing the initial dose of insulin in type 2 DM
HbA1C <8%
• Initial insulin dose = 0.1 to 0.2 units/ kg body wt
HbA1C > 8%
• Initial insulin dose = 0.2 to 0.3 units/ kg body wt

Initiation of insulin therapy as a single injection at bedtime is simple for the doctor and also more acceptable for the patient. Once FBS comes to acceptable value, then adjust the daytime oral agents to control daytime hyperglycemia while keeping the insulin dose constant. If daytime blood glucose levels become less, then decrease the dose of oral agents. Additional oral agents may be added to the existing oral agents, if daytime blood sugar is not adequately controlled.

Once Daily Insulin

Options for once daily insulin include the following:

- Once daily basal insulin (glargine or detemir or degludec)
- Once daily NPH
- Once daily premix insulin 30/70.

Twice Daily Insulin

Here a premix insulin (30/70 ratio) is added twice daily, one injection before breakfast and another injection before dinner. Oral agents can be continued along with this regimen.

Thrice Daily Insulin

Here short-acting insulin is given before breakfast and lunch, and a premix insulin is given before dinner (total 3 injections per day). Another regimen is to give premix insulin before every meal (total 3 injections).

Basal Bolus Regimen

Here short-acting insulin is given before every meal and a long acting basal injection is given at bedtime (total 4 injections per day).

The details of all these regimens are given in Chapter 5: Insulin Injection Regimens.

Further Dose Adjustments

Once the fasting blood sugar (FBS) is consistently in the desired range, then concentrate on prelunch, predinner and bed time blood sugar values. If these values are in the normal range it means that the daytime oral agents are acting. If these values are excessively low, then the dose of oral agents should be reduced. This happens because of decreased glucotoxicity by improved glucose control because of addition of insulin, leading to enhanced sensitivity to both oral agents and insulin. The dose of evening insulin should be kept constant while adjusting daytime oral agents. If the prelunch and predinnner blood glucose values are excessively high, then oral sulphonylureas are probably not contributing significantly to glycemic control. In such situation sulphonylureas can be discontinued and an insulin sensitizing agent like metformin or the glitazones can be added if the patient is not already on these agents. If the patient is already on all these oral agents on maximal doses, there may be no option left except to start two or more injections of insulin per day. Details on how to adjust insulin doses are given in subsequent chapters.

Benefits of Combining Oral Agent and Insulin

Achieves better glycemic control than insulin or oral agents used alone. It also improves lipid metabolism and suppresses hepatic glucose production. It can be started on OPD basis. Less total exogenous insulin is needed than with insulin alone thereby causing less weight gain and less peripheral hyperinsulinemia.

Chapter

5

Insulin Injection Regimens

Under basal conditions, the normal blood glucose concentration is maintained in a narrow range between 80 and 110 mg/dL because of a balance between glucose production and glucose utilization by peripheral tissues. Pancreas secretes continuous basal levels of 0.5 – 1 unit/hour of insulin (12 – 24 units/day), with increased secretions after meals.

An ideal insulin injection regimen should mimic this physiological insulin secretion. There should be a constant supply of basal insulin and also there should be provision of extra dose of insulin three times daily to take care of post-meal surge in glucose levels. In practice the constant basal level of insulin can be provided by a basal insulin (insulin glargine, detemir, or degludec). Post-meal glucose surge can be taken care by injecting insulin before every meal. This is called basal bolus insulin regimen and is the ideal one, but the problem is four injections per day which is worrisome for most patients. This basal bolus regimen can also be simulated by continuous subcutaneous insulin infusion (CSII) which eliminates the need for multiple insulin injections by using an insulin pump device. But everyone cannot afford CSII and the expertise to manage CSII is not available everywhere. Moreover the ideal basal bolus insulin regimen is required mainly in type 1 diabetes and advanced type 2 diabetes because in these two situations there is almost no insulin secretion from the pancreas. Hence, we need to supply both basal and meal related bolus dose of insulin. But for most other patients, there is some insulin secretion present in the body, and in such patients blood glucose can be controlled by one, or two, or three injections per day. So there are insulin injection regimens starting from one injection per day to multiple injections per day.

The basal component of insulin therapy has a prominent action on fasting blood glucose levels. Postprandial glycemia is taken care of by short-acting insulins given before each meal like lispro, aspart, glulisine, or regular insulin. Generally while trying to control FBS values, basal component of insulin should be adjusted and to control PPBS values, the short-acting component should be adjusted (with exception of twice daily mixed insulin regimen in which morning NPH has to be adjusted to control post lunch glycemia.

INSULIN REGIMENS FOR TREATMENT OF DIABETES

ONE INJECTION PER DAY

Most people with type 2 diabetes in the initial stages can be maintained on single dose of insulin per day because there is presence of some endogenous insulin secretion. Insulin can be added while continuing existing oral drugs. However, single injection of insulin per day may not work in type 1 diabetes where is no endogenous secretion of insulin. It is also not good for patients with advanced type 2 DM and pancreatic diabetes, where there is hardly any insulin secretion left.

Once Daily Basal Insulin (Best Option for Once Daily Regimen)

For patients for whom insulin is being started for the first time, it is better to start with once daily dose of basal insulin. It has better compliance and acceptance. Start at the dose of 10 units per day or 0.1 to 0.2 units/kg body weight per day. The total dose calculated is given once daily at bedtime. Basal insulin can also be given in the morning. Long acting basal insulins such as detemir or glargine or degludec are preferred over NPH because NPH does not act for 24 hours and has more risk of causing hypoglycemia especially if given at night (nocturnal hypoglycemia).

This basal insulin dose is adjusted by 10–15% or 2–4 units once or twice weekly to reach a target fasting plasma glucose (FPG).

If patient is already on some oral agents, these are continued as before. The rationale for combining oral agents with insulin is based on the assumption that if the night dose of basal insulin lowers FBS, then daytime oral agents will be more effective in controlling postprandial hyperglycemia and maintaining normal blood glucose levels throughout the day. Many studies have shown that fasting glucose contributes to daytime hyperglycemia. This high fasting blood glucose is because of hepatic glucose production, which can be decreased by night-time insulin.

Once Daily NPH

NPH insulin can also be given at bedtime to control FBS (not preferred). Giving NPH at bedtime is generally better than giving it in the morning before breakfast.

Once Daily Premix Insulin 30/70

A single dose of human premix insulin can be added to oral agents before dinner. This also has been shown to be an effective strategy in controlling blood sugars.

TWO INJECTIONS PER DAY

Most people obtain better sugar control using two or more injections of insulin per day. It is best to treat all patients with type 1 diabetes with two or more injections per day. An advanced stage of type 2 diabetes also requires 2 or more injections per day.

Mixtures of short-acting insulin (lispro, aspart, glulisine, regular) with intermediate acting insulin (NPH) can be used twice daily. Such mixtures are called biphasic insulins. Either they can be mixed just before injection or many premixed preparations are available in the market.

Twice-daily Injection of Mixed Insulin (Mixture of Short-Acting and Intermediate Insulin)

Study Fig. 5.1 given on the next page.

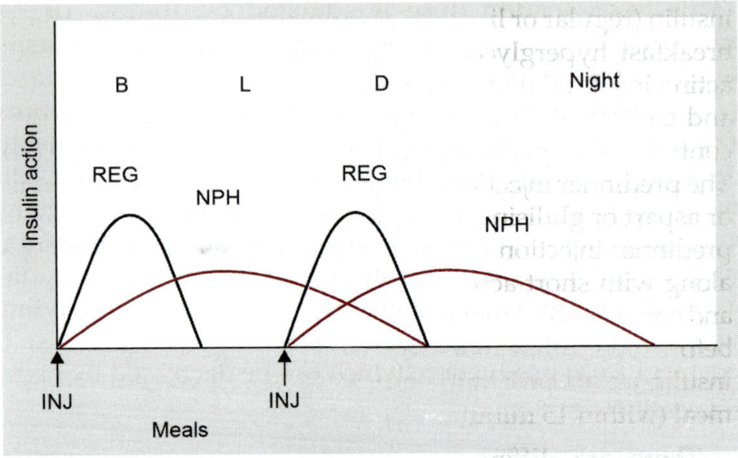

Fig. 5.1: Time–action profile of morning short-acting (regular) plus intermediate-acting insulin (NPH), predinner short-acting (regular) plus intermediate-acting insulin (NPH) B—Breakfast, L—Lunch, D—Dinner

This has been the most popular regimen until now because the number of injections given is only two per day. The short and intermediate acting insulins are either bought as separate bottles and mixed just before injecting or one of the premixed preparations available can be used. The advantage of using separate bottles is that both components can be adjusted independently thus allowing more flexibility and better control of hyperglycemia. However a significant number of patients experience difficulties with mixing intermediate- and short-acting insulin preparations because of an inability to mix insulin preparations in correct ratios or confusion between the different types of insulins. Such patients benefit from premixed preparations of short and intermediate acting insulin available in the market. Premixed preparations are available in the market in the ratio of 70:30, 50:50, or 75:25. The commonest premixed insulin used is human premix insulin 30/70 (30% short-acting and 70% NPH). These premixed insulins are convenient to use as there is no need to draw insulin from two different bottles (especially useful for people with poor vision) injections are given 30–40 minutes before breakfast and before dinner subcutaneously. The morning short-acting insulin (regular or lispro or aspart or glulisine) controls the post breakfast hyperglycemia. The peak of morning intermediate acting insulin (NPH) corresponds to post-lunch hyperglycemia and controls it. Thus, a single injection given before breakfast controls both post-breakfast and post-lunch hyperglycemia. The predinner injection of short-acting insulin (regular or lispro or aspart or glulisine) controls post-dinner hyperglycemia. The predinner injection of intermediate acting insulin (NPH) given along with short-acting insulin has its major action overnight and controls FBS. Human premix insulin has to be injected 30 min before food. Other analogue premix insulins such as aspart with insulin aspart protamine can be injected immediately before a meal (within 15 minutes of a meal).

There are differences in the pharmacokinetic and glucodynamic properties of 50/50 and 70/30 insulin premixes during the first 4 hours after injection, with significantly greater glucose lowering effect, higher insulin concentrations, and faster higher peaking after 50/50 injection. No significant differences were observed 4 hours after the insulin injections. This suggests that the risk for either late hypo- or hyperglycemia is unaffected by the type of insulin premix used. An other study directly comparing single injections of 50/50 and 70/30 insulin, reported significant differences between the two preparations in the first 4 h after a higher dose of insulin (0.3 units/kg). The exact clinical implications of these findings are yet to be clear. However, if the patients ratio of short and intermediate acting insulin matches one of the premixed preparation it can be used.

The combination of intermediate- and short-acting insulin in a two injections/day regimen is very often successful in type 2 diabetes. However, when high doses are used there may be midnight hypoglycemia (Somogyi phenomenon) and high FBS which commonly occurs in type 1 diabetes. It is less common in type 2 diabetes, probably because of differences in endogenous insulin secretory ability and intact counter regulatory mechanisms which prevent hypoglycemia.

As explained above, this regimen should potentially achieve normal basal, postprandial, and fasting blood sugars with just two injections per day. However, this regimen has many potential disadvantages. These are:

1. As explained in Fig. 5.1, the peak of morning intermediate acting insulin (NPH) occurs after lunch and before dinner and the peak of predinner NPH occurs after dinner somewhere in midnight (usually between 3 to 4 am). Therefore, if a high dose of NPH insulin is used in the morning, hypoglycemia may occur at midday especially if the lunch is delayed. Because of this, there is decreased flexibility to choose lunch timing and its quantity. Since the morning NPH has been given already, the patient cannot skip lunch or delay it, otherwise he will develop hypoglycemia. Patients may require a mid morning snack to avoid this problem. Similarly, the peaking of intermediate insulin action at midnight can cause nocturnal hypoglycemia.
2. Predinner NPH sometimes does not sustain its effect until morning and hence FBS may rise. Normally an increase in the dose of predinner NPH will control the high FBS. However, a very large dose of predinner NPH may peak in the midnight and produce hypoglycemia. A reactive hyperglycemia may result in the morning due to counter regulatory mechanisms trying to counteract midnight hypoglycemia (Somogyi phenomenon). This is where a common mistake happens. If you increase night NPH to control FBS, FBS values may paradoxically rise instead of falling. To avoid this, midnight (3 to 4 am) blood glucose should be measured while increasing the predinner NPH.
3. Another problem is that the action of morning NPH may get over by late afternoon and there may be no insulin coverage during this time until predinner injection given. This may result in high blood sugar levels before dinner. This happens especially in young and thin individuals because of rapid absorption and clearance of insulin.

Despite all these disadvantages, the twice-daily mixed insulin regimen remains popular. Infact, all the above disadvantages of this regimen may not be prominent in patients who still have some endogenous insulin secretion like in early stages of type 2 diabetes.

Twice-daily premixed insulin analogues (biphasic insulin lispro and biphasic insulin aspart)

Premixed insulin analogues combine rapid- and intermediate-acting insulin analogues. Studies have shown that, as compared with premixed human insulin, premixed insulin analogues result in better control of postprandial hyperglycemia, but no changes in glycosylated hemoglobin levels. Minor hypoglycemic events are same as that of premixed human insulin, but major hypoglycemic events are less compared to premixed human insulin.

THREE OR MORE INJECTIONS PER DAY

Those unable to achieve good sugar control with once or twice daily injection regimens may require three or more injections of insulin per day to achieve the same. In addition, most people using glargine, detemir, and degludec as their basal insulin need to take at least three injections per day.

Regimens requiring three or more shots per day are:

- *Before breakfast*: Premixed human insulin or premixed insulin analogue
- *Before dinner*: Short-acting insulin (regular or lispro or aspart or glulisine)
- *Before dinner/bedtime:* NPH or long acting basal insulin (glargine or detemir or degludec) OR
- *Before each meal:* Regular or lispro or aspart or glulisine
- Morning or night (before dinner/bedtime): Glargine or detemir

Premixed Insulin before Breakfast, Short-acting Insulin before Dinner and Intermediate-acting Insulin at Bedtime

One popular solution to the problem of midnight hypoglycemia and morning hyperglycemia which is because of peaking of NPH at midnight and no action in the morning is to delay the injection of predinner NPH to a later time, i.e. do not give NPH before dinner, give it at bedtime (but give short-acting insulin before dinner as before). Details of this regimen are explained as follows.

Study Fig. 5.2 given on the next page.

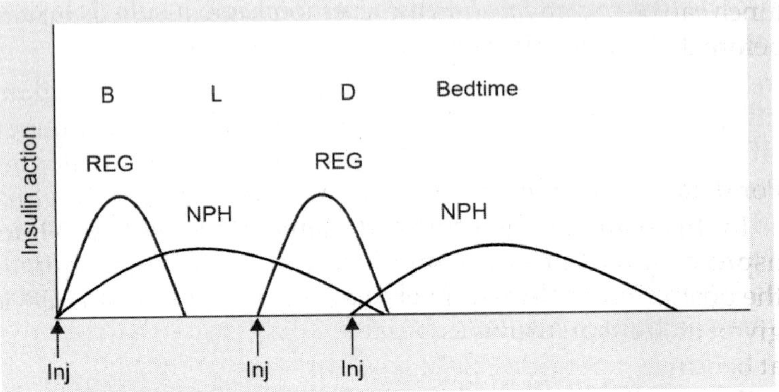

Fig. 5.2: Time–action profile of premix insulin before breakfast, predinner short-acting insulin and bedtime intermediate-acting insulin

Total number of injections in this regimen becomes 3.

Delaying night NPH to bedtime makes its peak correspond to early morning, the time when it is actually needed (because of increase in growth hormone and corticosteroids which cause early morning increase in blood sugar) thus avoiding midnight hypoglycemia and controlling morning hyperglycemia.

Smaller dose of NPH is required when injected at bedtime (at 10 to 11 pm) than what would be required if the NPH were to be given before dinner. This is because it has to last only for 8 to 9 hr, since it is injected late. Exact dose required should be decided based on FBS values. The advantage of bedtime NPH has been shown in many studies in decreasing nocturnal hypoglycemia and improving fasting hyperglycemia.

However, the decreased flexibility of lunch timing and its quantity remains with this regimen due to the use of premix insulin before breakfast. NPH component in premix insulin given before breakfast controls post-lunch hyperglycemia. Hence, the quantity and timing of lunch should be consistent everyday. This problem can be overcome by using basal bolus regimen which consists of 3 short-acting insulin injections before breakfast, lunch and dinner and NPH at bedtime, a total of 4 injections. Since short-acting insulin is given before each meal, there is flexibility in meal timings and quantity. For example, lunch can be had any time in the afternoon, and insulin is injected before that meal. This regimen is explained below.

Short-acting Insulin before Each Meal (3 Injections) and NPH or long-acting Insulin at Bedtime (1 Injection)

For details shown in **Fig. 5.3**.

In this regimen, the short-acting insulin (regular insulin or lispro or aspart or glulisine) given before each meal controls the postprandial glucose levels and NPH or long acting insulin given at bedtime provides basal insulin level. If NPH is given at bedtime, it provides basal level throughout the night. If long acting insulin (glargine, detemir, degludec) is given at bedtime, it provides basal insulin throughout the day. The bedtime dose of NPH can also be given with predinner short-acting insulin if there is no significant risk of nocturnal hypoglycemia and FBS control does not deteriorate. The main advantage of this regimen as explained earlier is the greater flexibility of meals.

When insulin lispro or aspart or glulisine is used as prandial insulin, there may be windows of absent or less insulin levels as the action of these insulins gets over fast. This situation may arise in type 1 DM and advanced type 2 DM when there

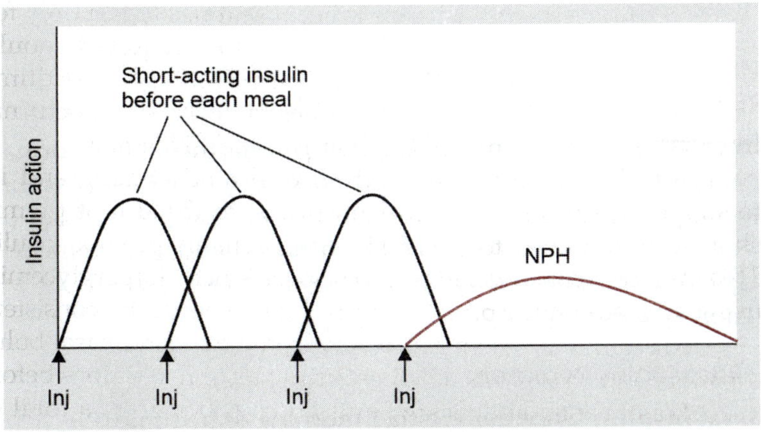

Fig. 5.3: Time–action profile of short-acting insulin (REG) before each meal and basal intermediate-acting insulin at bedtime

is little endogenous insulin secretion to provide continuous basal levels of insulin. This happens towards the end of insulin action and corresponds to a time period before the meals. In such situations NPH has to be given twice daily. A small dose of NPH in the morning and a larger dose at bedtime, provides continuous basal insulin throughout the day. This may not be a problem with regular human insulin as it has slightly longer duration of action than the new rapid acting insulin analogues. However, due to the availability of long acting once daily basal insulins such as glargine, detemir, and degludec, twice daily NPH is rarely used now.

Premix Insulin Three Times Daily before Every Meal

Many studies have shown that thrice daily injection of premix insulin before each meal is more efficacious in reducing HbA1c level in patients who are poorly controlled on twice daily premix insulin. Studies have been done using thrice daily biphasic insulin aspart (BIAsp) and thrice daily biphasic insulin lispro. Studies have been done using human biphasic insulin also with similar results.

Hence before going for basal bolus regimen which usually requires 4 injections per day, thrice daily premix insulin can be an option. Time action profile of this regimen is shown in **Fig. 5.4**.

MULTIPLE INJECTION REGIMENS USING BASAL BOLUS REGIMENS (INTENSIVE INSULIN REGIMENS)

Intensive insulin regimens attempt to mimic the body's normal pattern of insulin secretion, and make use of a basal insulin to supply a constant level of basal insulin and bolus doses of short-acting insulin to cover the meal related requirements. This can be achieved either by basal bolus regimens or by using an insulin pump.

Basal Bolus Regimen

Basal insulin: Once daily, either morning or bedtime **(Fig. 5.5)**. Preferred basal insulin is glargine or detemir or degludec. Alternative is NPH given two times morning and bedtime.

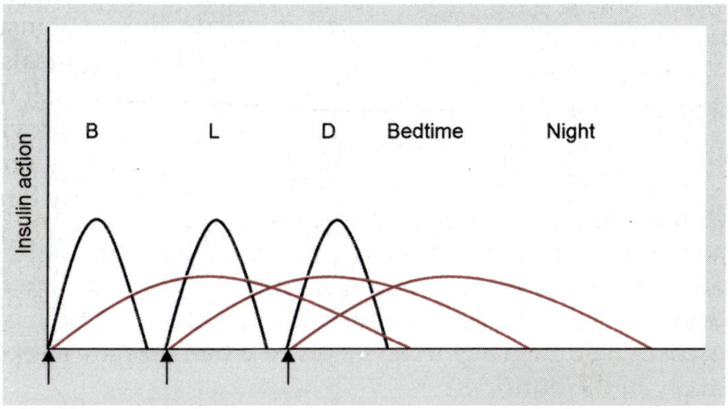

Fig. 5.4: Premix insulin injection given before each meal (black—short-acting insulin, blue—intermediate-acting insulin)

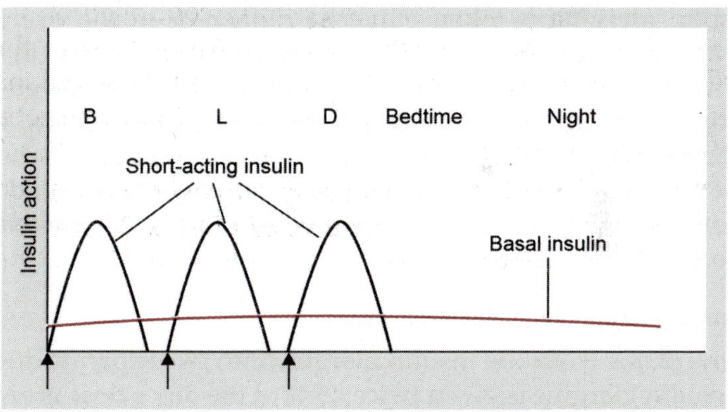

Fig. 5.5: Basal bolus regimen (black—short-acting insulin, blue—long-acting e.g. insulin)

Bolus insulin: Fast acting insulin (lispro or aspart or glulisine) is preferred before each meal. Alternatively regular insulin may be used.

Regimens Using Glargine as Basal Insulin

Insulin glargine with short-acting insulin (regular or lispro or aspart of glulisine)

Insulin glargine is taken in the evening or night (6 to 10 pm) and short-acting insulin (regular or lispro or aspart or glulisine) is taken before each meal. The advantage of taking insulin glargine at 6 to10 pm is that its activity can decrease after 20–24 hours. This is the time (6 to 10 pm) when the dinner short-acting insulin is working, and so the decrease does not matter. If the activity of insulin glargine lessens after 20 hours, the dinner short-acting insulin will cover this time period.

Insulin glargine and short-acting insulin (regular or lispro or aspart or glulisine) can both be given at dinner time. But they should not be mixed together and must be given in separate syringes or pens. For infants or those who have trouble with injections, insulin glarginecan be given when they are sleeping (usually in the buttocks).

Insulin glargine at night, premix insulin before breakfast and short-acting insulin before dinner

Insulin glargine is taken either at dinner or in the evening as above. A mixture of NPH and short-acting insulin (in the same syringe) is taken prior to breakfast. This works well for people who do not want to take an afternoon injection, like children who are not ready to take a noon injection at school. The morning NPH insulin will help to cover lunch and an afternoon snack also if any. One dose of short-acting insulin is injected before dinner.

Insulin glargine divided as two doses

Some prefer to divide insulin glargine into two separate doses. If insulin glargine is given twice, 25% of the day's dose is given in the morning and 75% in the night. This may involve five shots of insulin per day, including injections of short-acting insulin before each meal. Dividing insulin glargine dose in this way may give more insulin activity during the daytime since more insulin is required during daytime.

Initial dose of insulin glargine

The dosage of insulin glargine should be determined individually for each patient based on blood glucose levels and previous insulin therapy. Generally, in a type 2 diabetic patient who is not already receiving any insulin, insulin glargine can be started at 10 units once daily. Dosage is then adjusted based on the patient's blood glucose levels. In patients who are already receiving once daily NPH insulin, the same number of units is given as insulin glargine. However, if a patient is receiving twice daily NPH insulin, then the dosage of insulin glargine is reduced by approximately 20% for the first week of treatment and then adjusted according to blood glucose values. Monitoring of blood glucose may be necessary during the change of insulins and during early weeks of therapy. If the patient can monitor his blood glucose values himself (at least 4 to 5 times/day) using glucometer, this is also ok.

The dosage and timing of additional short-acting insulin or oral antidiabetic agents may need to be adjusted. Dose adjustments of both insulin and oral antidiabetic drugs may be required when there is change in patient's body weight or lifestyle, and during intercurrent illness. As with all subcutaneous insulin injections, the site should be rotated within an area after each injection. To avoid hypoglycemia, elderly patients require cautious dose selection and titration. Consideration should also be given to any other drug that the patient is taking which may affect glycemic control. Appropriate caution should be taken in renal or liver impairment and the dose of insulin glargine is reduced as appropriate.

A useful rule of thumb is to start glargine at half the total units of intermediate-acting insulin taken per day. *For example,* if 40 units of NPH insulin was being taken in the morning and 20 units were being taken at dinner, a total of 60 units of intermediate-acting insulin was taken per day. Then start the person on 30 units of insulin glargine insulin. This dose can then be titrated based on FBS values.

Timing of Insulin Glargine Injection

Most large studies of type 2 diabetes that evaluated insulin glargine without prandial insulin were performed with the use of bedtime injections. However, one large study involving 695 subjects with type 2 diabetes reported greater reductions in glycosylated hemoglobin levels with morning injections of insulin glargine than with bedtime injections (both groups also received glimepiride in the morning). Similarly, in 378 subjects with type 1 diabetes who received once-daily insulin glargine and prandial insulin lispro, the 24-hour glucose profiles were identical, regardless of whether the basal insulin was injected at breakfast, dinner, or bedtime. However, emerging data suggest that the provision of a once-daily dose of insulin glargine as the basal insulin may not be effective for all patients with severe insulin deficiency, particularly those with type1 diabetes.

Most studies involving insulin glargine have compared it with NPH insulin. Most trials have shown no differences or occasional improvements in glycemic control with insulin glargine. Most of the trials have shown that compared to NPH insulin, glargine is associated with decreased risk of hypoglycemia, especially nocturnal hypoglycemia.

Regimens using Detemir as Basal Insulin

Detemir is a basal insulin analogue and is well tolerated by both type 1 and type 2 diabetes patients. It is an option as basal component in basal-bolus insulin therapy. Clinical studies have shown better control of FBS with detemir than NPH.

Once daily bedtime administration of detemir with mealtime short-acting insulin

Once daily injection of detemir is usually given at bedtime. Regular insulin, lispro or aspart can be used as mealtime insulins.

Twice daily detemir with mealtime short-acting insulins

Detemir can also be given twice daily. When given twice daily steady serum levels are reached after 2–3 injections. The night dose of detemir can be given either before dinner or at bedtime.

Clinical efficacy of detemir based regimens

Most of the trials have compared detemir with NPH insulin and almost all have shown that detemir leads to more predictable blood sugar control with less risk of hypoglycemia and less weight gain. However, there is no significant improvement of HbA1c levels than that provided by NPH. A six and half months trial involving 347 patients and another 4 months trial with 140 patients did not show any significant difference in HbA1c levels at end point, though there was better control of FBS with detemir than NPH. A meta-analysis of 6 multinational trials involving both type 1 and type 2 diabetes patients comparing detemir and NPH insulin found improved glycemic control with detemir than NPH (mean HbA1c 7.79 with detemir and 7.88 with NPH). Almost all the trials have shown less variability in FBS levels with detemir. Greater predictability of insulin detemir implies that a better balance between glycemic control and hypoglycemic risk may be achievable.

Glargine vs Detemir as Basal Insulin

Most studies demonstrate a relatively peak-less action of both glargine and detemir and a comparable duration of action that is dose-dependent. Both glargine and detemir are equally effective and suitable for once daily injection to achieve glycemic control. Safety and efficacy profiles are similar for both, with less hypoglycemia compared with NPH. Insulin glargine has a greater affinity for the human IGF-1 receptor and greater mitogenic potential, compared with human insulin and detemir, but further studies are needed to determine the clinical significance ofthis. Considering all these, there is no real advantage of one over the other and choosing between glargine and detemir comes down to personal preference and patient preferences. When higher dose of basal insulin is required, glargine may be preferable as it has almost flat profile of action than detemir. At higher doses detemir may have to be split into two doses and given in the morning and night. One meta-analysis showed that to achieve the same glycaemic control insulin detemir was often injected twice daily in a higher dose but with less weight gain, while insulin glargine was only injected once daily, with somewhat fewer injection site reactions.

Degludec as Basal Insulin

Degludec is an ultra long-acting basal insulin (longer duration of action than glargine and detemir). Degludec has flat and stable glucose-lowering profile, a duration of action exceeding 30 h and less inter-patient variation in glucose-lowering effect than insulin glargine. Many studies have shown that compared with glargine, degludec is associated with equivalent HbA1c control and significantly lower nocturnal hypoglycemia rates.

Degludec is also associated with significantly greater reductions in FBS and lower total doses of insulin versus glargine.

In addition, there is more flexibility in the time of degludec administration. It can be injected at bedtime or anytime of the day without compromising glycemic control.

One major advantage of degludec is it can be mixed with short-acting insulin and injected as one injection. The chemical properties of insulin degludec have allowed the development of a soluble co-formulation with prandial insulin aspart (insulin degludec/insulin aspart). This brings down the number of injections to three (instead of four) in basal bolus regimens using degludec as basal insulin. This advantage is not there with glargine and detemir which cannot be mixed with any short-acting insulin.

Insulin Analogues vs Conventional Insulins

- Compared with conventional human insulin, use of the analogues was associated with a small decrease in HbA1c levels in type 1 diabetics but not type 2 diabetics.
- Use of an analogue did not reduce the overall frequency of hypoglycemia compared with human insulin in either type 1 or type 2 diabetics.
- However, severe hypoglycemia occurred less often with the analogues than with human insulin.
- None of the studies were designed to assess the possible long-term benefits or safety of the short-acting insulin analogues.

Monitoring Blood Sugars during Insulin Therapy

Initially while adjusting insulin, blood glucose should be ideally measured before every meal, 1–2 hours after every meal, at bedtime and at 3 am (8 times per day) until the achievement of normal blood sugar values. After this the recommended frequency is daily fasting glucose plus 1 to 3 other samples (mostly preprandial or bedtime) on most days, with a complete profile (7 or more determinations) weekly. Patient should ideally continue with 3 to 4 daily measurements (preprandial and bedtime).

For pregnant patients, 4 to 8 measurements daily are necessary, with complete profile obtained at least 1 to 2 times weekly. For stable patients with type 2 diabetes, fasting samples should be measured 3 to 7 times weekly, with a complete profile (7–8 samples) 1 to 3 times monthly. If hypoglycemia is suspected any time additional samples should be drawn at that time. Frequent sampling may also be necessary during inter current illness.

These recommendations are from American Diabetic Association (ADA). ADA also recommends that the frequency of blood glucose monitoring be individualized. Obviously, such a frequency of measurements is possible only if the patient himself does the measurements using glucometer. This is called self-monitoring of blood glucose (SMBG). SMBG is a part and parcel of insulin therapy. These measurements are done either by the patient himself using glucometer or with the help of a health care provider. Frequent SMBG is mandatory in pregnant patients. Desired glycemic control can be obtained through SMBG without frequent, prolonged, or expensive hospital admissions. SMBG is obligatory in all patients who are using a portable insulin infusion pump. SMBG also helps to rule out nocturnal hypoglycemia.

HbA1C should be measured approximately every 3 months in all diabetic patients. HbA1C measurement provides an index of glycemic status over the previous 2 to 3 months. Expert opinion recommends at least 2 measurements per year for those meeting treatment goals and has stable glycemic control.

Glycated serum protein (GSP): Because the turnover of human albumin is much shorter (half-life 14 to 20 days) than Hb (erythrocyte life span is 120 days), measurements of total GSP and GSA (glycated serum albumin) provide an index of glycemic status over the preceding 1 to 2 weeks. Measurement of GSP is useful in situations where HbA1C cannot be measured like hemolytic anemias where RBC life span is reduced and Hb turnover is very high. Measurement of GSP should not be considered equivalent to the HbA1C test, since it only indicates glycemic control over a short time. GSP assays need to be performed on a monthly basis to gather the same information provided by the HbA1C test performed 3 to 4 times a year. Unlike the HbA1C, GSP has not been shown to correlate with the development or progression of complications of diabetes.

Intensive Diabetes Therapy

Intensive diabetes therapy can minimize diabetes related morbidity and mortality. It needs some amount of commitment from the patient and his family side.

Components Intensive Diabetes Therapy

1. Multiple component insulin regimen
2. Balance of food intake, activity, and insulin dose
3. Daily SMBG (self monitoring of blood glucose)
4. Use of predetermined algorithms to adjust food intake or supplemental insulin
5. Individualized target blood glucose levels
6. Frequent contact between patient and doctor
7. Patient education and motivation
8. Psychological support
9. Objective assessment (glycosylated hemoglobin)

All these components were used on patients participating in DCCT and UKPDS trials. The goals for diabetes control need to be individualized based on a patient's situation. For example, an HbA1C of 7% may be reasonable in a 20 years old college student, but for a 30 years old pregnant lady, this would be 6%. Many patients above 50 years of age may not need strict glycemic control. However, it should be attempted in all patients where appropriate.

All the patients on intensive diabetes therapy should maintain the following:

Basic activity plan: Should be kept relatively constant. Unusual exercise requires changes in food intake or change in insulin dosage or both. Different activity plans such as weekend versus weekday, summer versus winter, etc. may require adjustment of diet and/or dosage of insulin.

Basic meal plan: Food intake must be relatively consistent from day to day in terms of calories and composition. Rapidly absorbed simple sugars should be omitted from the basic daily meal. Any change in food may require adjustment of insulin dosage and/or activity.

Regular and frequent monitoring of blood glucose: Blood glucose levels should be checked regularly in order to adjust diet, exercise, drugs, and insulin dosages. Glycosylated hemoglobin should be checked once in 4 to 8 weeks to document the control attained.

Patients and his family should be educated in all aspects of diabetes care. Psychological counseling of the patient and the family may be necessary as the patient himself and his family may be having psychological stress after the diagnosis of diabetes.

Chapter

6

New Methods of Insulin Delivery

CONTINUOUS SUBCUTANEOUS INSULIN INFUSION

Continuous subcutaneous insulin infusion (CSII) also known as insulin pump is an effective means of implementing intensive insulin therapy in both type I and type 2 diabetes. It can achieve near normal levels of blood glucose and provide improved flexibility of lifestyle.

In CSII buffered regular insulin or rapid acting insulin analogues are used (lispro or aspart or glulisine). Insulin is infused continuously in microlitre amounts along with prandial bolus infusions. It is done through a catheter attached to an insulin pump which is worn externally. The catheter is connected to a transcutaneous needle or silastic infusion set. Silastic infusion set is placed into the subcutaneous tissue with the help of a needle and needle is then removed. This provides more comfort for the patients, though chances of kinking are also more. Currently available insulin pumps are small in size and easy to use. The syringe, catheter and skin site setup are changed by the patient every 2 to 3 days and sometimes after a longer period. CSII therapy is more expensive than multiple injections.

Studies have shown that rapid acting insulin analogues provide better control of blood sugar than regular insulin. Lispro is quickly replacing buffered regular insulin in this regard. Use of insulin mixtures in pumps has not been studied and is not recommended.

Where to use:

- Traditionally, CSII has been used mainly in type 1 diabetes patients. Insulin pumps may be considered in all pediatric patients with type 1 diabetes, especially those children under 7 years of age (Fig. 6.1).

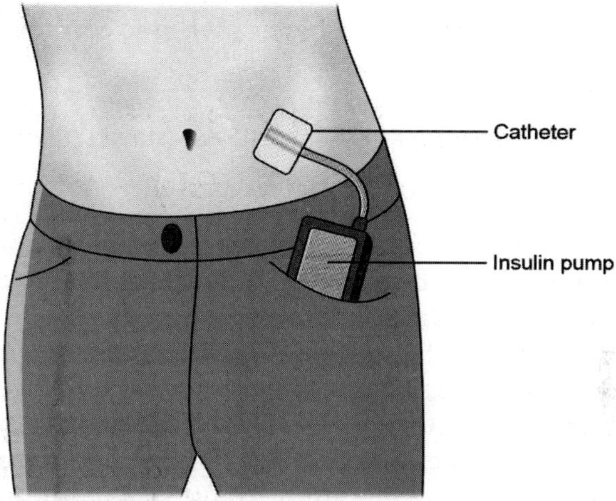

Fig. 6.1: Continuous subcutaneous insulin infusion

- In type 2 diabetics who have not achieved glycemic control with multiple subcutaneous injections.
- It can also be used instead of multiple injections in both type 1 and type 2 diabetics, especially those who desire more flexible lifestyle.
- People who have insulin allergy do well with CSSI as continuous delivery of insulin suppresses allergic reactions rather than intermittent delivery.
- Any motivated patient wishing to improve glycemic control especially those on multiple injections with poor sugar control.
- **Pregnancy:** In pregnancy complicated by diabetes, CSII compared to MDI (multiple dose injections) gives better glycemic control; this difference is more in first trimester, but decreases in subsequent trimesters. CSII therapy is also associated with lower insulin requirements. Infants from the CSII group are more likely to be large for gestational age and less likely to be small for gestational age. Various rapid acting insulin analogues used in insulin pumps have been found to be safe during pregnancy.

- People with extreme insulin sensitivity and frequent hypoglycemia can achieve better glycemic control with less chances of hypoglycemia.
- Hypoglycemia unawareness.
- Severe early morning insulin resistance (dawn phenomenon).

Advantages of CSII

Because of the more physiologic delivery of insulin, good glycemic control may be achieved with lesser insulin than that needed for multiple daily injections.

- RCTs comparing CSII and multiple subcutaneous injections with insulin analogs have shown modest improvement in A1C in type 1 diabetes. However, in type 2 diabetes, reduction in A1C has not been better than multiple subcutaneous injections, although a few studies have shown improvement.
- There is also evidence that CSII may reduce DKA risk and diabetes complications, particularly retinopathy and peripheral neuropathy in youth, compared with MDI.
- There is reduction of hypoglycemic events.
- Insulin pump therapy allows increased flexibility in meal timing and meal quantity and also increased flexibility in the time and intensity of exercise.
- Better quality of life in terms of self reliance and control.
- Insulin pump therapy allows consistent insulin absorption and pharmakokinetic profile resulting in reduced fluctuations and better glycemic control.

Disadvantages of CSII

Some disadvantages of CSII compared to MDI include extra cost and supervision. There is also a risk of pump malfunction, catheter occlusion leading to chances of DKA. Catheter insertion site infections can occur though rare.

Automated Insulin Delivery (AID) Systems

AID systems increase and decrease insulin delivery based on sensor-derived glucose levels. These systems consist of three components—an insulin pump, a continuous glucose sensor, and an algorithm that determines insulin delivery.

Sensor-Augmented Pumps

Sensor-augmented pumps that suspend insulin when glucose is low or predicted to go low within the next 30 min have been approved by the FDA. These devices have been shown to reduce hypoglycemia events especially nocturnal hypoglycemia events.

CONTINUOUS INTRAPERITONEAL INSULIN INFUSION (CIPII)

Continuous intraperitoneal insulin infusion (CIPII) is intended to enable the infusion of insulin into the peritoneal cavity. The main advantage of this method is that it more closely resembles the physiological insulin secretion than the other conventional therapies because it goes to liver first just like insulin secreted from pancreas. The insulin delivery catheter is inserted into the peritoneal cavity. The catheter is placed through the rectus sheath and floats freely in the peritoneal cavity. The insulin pump can either be implanted under the subcutaneous fat just above the rectus sheath in the abdominal area or the pump can be kept externally.

A trial by Veterans affairs cooperative studies with type 2 diabetes patients, who had previously not responded to other insulin regimens, compared intraperitoneal with multiple daily subcutaneous insulin injections. There was almost equal improvement in glycemic control and HbA1C levels to near normal levels. However, there were many advantages with intraperitoneal insulin. There was reduced incidence of hypoglycemia and decreased weight gain. The superior pharmacokinetics of intraperitoneal insulin was also demonstrated in another trial by Kelly, et al. This study showed rapid peak and rapid clearance of insulin within 2 to 3 hr. The glucose disposal rate was also higher.

Although the reduction in HbA1c levels by CIPII treatment is limited, the fact that such an improvement can be achieved simply by switching the site of insulin delivery is noteworthy, especially as the total daily insulin dose remains unchanged, combined with a reduction in the frequency of severe hypoglycemia compared to CSII.

Problems with CIPII are risk of catheter occlusion, pump malfunction, and peritoneal infection.

ORAL INSULIN (HEXYL INSULIN)

Oral delivery of insulin is one of the most promising and anticipated areas in the treatment of diabetes, because it avoids the need for insulin injections and significantly improves the quality of life of diabetics. Another advantage of oral insulin delivery is that it passes through the liver first before reaching systemic circulation which is similar to physiological insulin secretion.

The main problem with oral insulin is that the insulin molecule is too large to get through the membrane in the gut or is degraded there by digestive enzymes. Newer technologies to prevent insulin degradation in the GIT and to facilitate its absorption are under trial. These include insulin capsules coated with trypsin inhibitor, insulin loaded on to nanoparticles to liposomes, self-emulsifying systems, and hydrogels. Many of these newer technologies are under trial and have shown promising results in preliminary studies.

It will still take some time for oral insulins formulations to come out of all the limitations and become the standard therapy.

BUCCAL INSULIN

Generex Biotechnology Corporation is developing a device, which looks like the metered dose inhalers used by asthmatics, but it has been modified so that Oral-Lyn, a liquid aerosol version of insulin, is absorbed by the mucous membranes in the cheeks, tongue, and throat. Research done by the company showed that the effect of Oral-Lyn was similar to insulin injection in its ability to lower blood glucose levels. Further, Oral-Lyn was able to serve as the mealtime boost needed by some people who are failing on oral hypoglycemic drugs. However, Oral-Lyn trial has been delayed and the final phase is not yet completed. Another molecule being developed by Shreya Life Sciences Pvt. Ltd. India is oral Recosulin® and the results of the phase 2 and phase 3 trials are awaited. Another formulation "insulin loaded orally dissolved films" is undergoing investigation.

INHALED INSULIN (INTRAPULMONARY)

Inhaled insulin is a novel method of insulin delivery. When introduced to the market in 2006, in halable insulin was considered a significant innovation to address needle phobia and incorrect insulin injection techniques. The liquid insulin is contained in a pellet, which is vaporized in an inhaler, aerosolizing the liquid insulin. Inhaled insulin can also be delivered as a dry powder inhaled through a mouthpiece. Inhaled insulin is more rapidly absorbed than subcutaneous insulin. Hence, this route may be appropriate for the administration of pre-meal insulin. Many trials have already been done with inhaled insulin and have shown improved postprandial sugar control. However, there was increased risk of hypoglycemia.

Inhaled insulin has been observed to produce greater antibody response than subcutaneously injected insulin. This antibody response was more common in type 1 than type 2 diabetic patients. Peak antibody response is generally observed 6–12 months after therapy. However, there was no increased incidence of allergy or other hypersensitivity reactions. Inhaled insulin did not produce any deterioration of pulmonary function tests except occasional cough. Hypoglycemia and weight gain were observed as expected with other insulin preparations. Pulmonary function tests were not altered in any of the studies except mild cough.

However, insulin inhaler devices have not found commercial success so far and are not popular because of safety concerns, and competing products.

THE SKIN PATCH

The main problem with transdermal insulin delivery is stratum corneum which acts as a barrier to insulin absorption. There are several techniques to overcome this barrier, such as iontophoresis (uses small electric currents to vaporize stratum corneum), sonophereis or phonopheresis (uses ultrasound waves), microdermal ablation (removes stratum corneum, electroporation (utilizes high voltage pulses that are applied for a very short time), transfersulin (insulin encapsulated in transferosome, an elastic, flexible vesicle which squeeze by itself to deliver drugs through skin pores), InsuPatch™, a device developed as an add-on to an insulin pump that applies local heat to the skin in order to increase the absorption of insulin.

All these techniques are still under trial and have not yet come into mass market.

Chapter

7

Insulin Dose Adjustments

Adjustment of insulin requires some thinking and basic knowledge about the time action profiles of different insulin preparations. Insulin adjustment is a dynamic and ongoing process. Insulin dose adjustments are made based on frequent blood sugar measurements. There are some basic principles, which should be adhered to while adjusting insulin doses.

Insulin dose adjustments can be:

- Basic dose adjustments, which will be followed daily
- Temporary adjustments, e.g. during illness, change in activity or change in meals

The total required dose of insulin per day to control hyperglycemia in a patient with stable food and activity pattern is called "basic" insulin dose. Successful implementation of insulin therapy requires co-operation from the patient to pay careful attention to meal planning, activity, and blood glucose monitoring. Target blood sugar goals should be individualized depending on the patient's age, ability to recognize and recover from hypoglycemia, pregnancy, etc. For relatively young and healthy patients, who are able to recognize and respond to hypoglycemia a near normal glycemic control should be the target.

Choosing the Initial Dose of Insulin for Type 1 DM Patients

The insulin dose required for a type 1 diabetic patient, within 20% of their ideal body weight in the absence of intercurrent infection or other periods of instability, approximates 0.4 to 1 unit/kg/day. During periods of relative remission ("honeymoon period") during which beta-cell activity may increase, requirements may be less. During periods of intercurrent illness, insulin requirements may be high. Requirement is also high during adolescent growth spurt.

In general, the total initial dose per day in type 1 DM patients = 0.4 to 0.1 units per kg body.

Choosing the Initial Total Dose of Insulin for Type 2 DM Patients

If HbA1C <8%

- Initial insulin dose = 0.1 to 0.2 units/ kg body wt

If HbA1C >8%

- Initial insulin dose = 0.2 to 0.3 units/ kg body wt

Distribution of Total Required Insulin Dose Throughout the Day

Initial insulin distribution is empirically chosen as follows. However, there are no hard and fast rules for this. Distribution may be changed based on individual cases. Various components of insulin are then adjusted to achieve the desired glycemic control **(Table 7.1)**.

Table 7.1: Distribution of total required insulin dose throughout the day

Regimen	*Insulin distribution*
Once daily injection: Basal insulin added to oral agents	Start with 5 to 10 units once daily at bedtime (0.1 to 0.2 units/kg/daily)
Twice daily premix insulin (short acting + intermediate acting insulin regimen) (premixed insulins are available in the ratio of 70:30, 75:25 and 50:50)	Give 2/3rds of mixture in the morning, and 1/3rd in the night
Regular plus intermediate before breakfast, regular before dinner, intermediate at bedtime	Distribution is same as above. Only difference is intermediate acting insulin is given at bedtime
3 injections of premix	1/3 before breakfast; 1/3 before lunch; 1/3 before dinner
4 injection daily, i.e. short acting insulin before each meal and intermediate insulin at bedtime	25% as short-acting insulin before breakfast 25% as short-acting insulin before lunch

Contd...

Contd...

Regimen	*Insulin distribution*
	25% as short-acting insulin before dinner 25% of the total daily dose given at bedtime as intermediate acting insulin
Basal bolus regimens: Long-acting insulin once daily as basal insulin (glargine or detemir or degludec) Short-acting insulin before each meal (regular or lispro or aspart or glulisine)	40% of the total as basal insulin. Remaining 60% is divided equally and given before each meal as short-acting insulin
Continuous subcutaneous insulin infusion	40% as continuous basal infusion 20% as pre breakfast bolus 20% as pre lunch bolus 20% as pre dinner bolus

Insulin distributions as above are just general guidelines. You can modify the percentages depending on the individual patients. Unusual meal pattern may need a deviation from the above scheme. Note that the premeal injection of short acting insulin has to be given 20–30 minutes before each meal if you are using regular insulin or just before meals if you are using lispro or aspart or glulisine.

ADJUSTMENT OF INSULIN DOSE

When glucose values are outside the target range consistently, adjustments are made in the insulin dosage. Adjustments may be temporary as in case of intercurrent illness and stress. Make sure that the high blood glucose levels are not caused by unusual change in food intake or physical activity. One important thing before adjusting the night dose insulin to lower FBS is to make sure that the midnight glucose levels (between 3 to 4 am especially for NPH) are not in the hypoglycemic range (i.e. not below 60 mg/dL). Caution is required before increasing night dose of insulin to correct high FBS, which in fact may be a rebound phenomenon due to midnight hypoglycemia (Somogyi phenomenon). Generally, adjustments are based on the following guidelines:

- The FBS values are brought under control by adjusting basal component of insulin (with the caveat as noted above)
- The postprandial glycemia is brought under control by adjusting the meal related component of insulin (this means adjusting the premeal short-acting insulin except in twice daily mixed insulin regimen where morning intermediate-acting insulin is adjusted to control post-lunch glucose levels).
- Before adjusting the meal related components see that the premeal blood glucose levels are within the acceptable range, if not take one or more of the following actions:
  - Decrease carbohydrate from the previous meal and add more fiber to that meal
  - Alter the timing of premeal insulin administration (give a longer interval between the injection and meal)
  - Increase the insulin dose given before the previous meal, (add an intervening snack if hypoglycemia is a risk)
- The overall insulin sensitivity of an individual will determine the amount of insulin required to correct a high blood sugar reading. One unit of regular insulin may result in a blood glucose drop of 100 mg/dL in a very insulin sensitive person, whereas only 25 mg/dL drop may be seen in a insulin resistant person. An average response would be 40–50 mg/dL decrement. Usually the more elevated the glucose, the more insulin is needed to bring it back to normal. The presence of ketones or acidosis requires even higher doses of insulin. Hence, the increments of insulin while adjusting should be 1 to 2 units at a time. However, in patients weighing >50 kg, during the period of initial stabilization, increments may be up to 3 to 4 units if the blood glucose value exceeds the target range by 100 mg/dL or more.
- Increments in each insulin component are made every 2 to 3 days. Allowing 2 to 3 days gap between adjustments will help in stabilizing the action of insulin and also helps in the confirmation of elevated glucose levels by allowing time for 2 to 3 measurements.

- Adjust only one insulin component at a time, beginning with the component responsible for controlling FBS, except when there is extreme hyperglycemia (>200 mg/dL) throughout the day signifying gross insulin deficiency. In that case, all the insulin components may need simultaneous adjustment. After FBS is brought under control, other insulin components should be adjusted starting with pre-breakfast short-acting insulin (regular or lispro or aspart). Once post-breakfast glucose levels are under control (confirm this by measuring 1 to 2 hours post-breakfast glucose values and pre-lunch glucose values), then adjust pre-lunch insulin dosage to control post-lunch blood glucose levels. Once this is under control next move on to pre-dinner insulin adjustment to control post-dinner glycemia. In this way glycemic control is gradually attained. Detailed algorithms for doing this are given in the following pages.
- Whenever there are symptoms suggestive of hypoglycemia, it should be verified by checking blood sugar level whenever possible. This will exclude other causes like anxiety, syncope etc as the cause of symptoms. When hypoglycemia is documented, or strongly suspected, it should be treated with a rapidly absorbed sugar or if the patient is in altered sensorium by giving 50 ml of 50% glucose intravenously. Patients should keep a source of readily available sugar with them always. If mealtime is more than one hour away, an additional slowly absorbed carbohydrate should be consumed (or protein). Hypoglycemia episodes are often readily explainable by known alterations in food or activity (e.g. a delayed meal or change in physical activity). If such is the case, there is no need to alter the existing insulin dose. If such is not the case, then the relevant insulin component responsible for hypoglycemia should be reduced by 1 to 2 units the next day. A one-off, high glucose level is not likely to be problematic, but even one episode of hypoglycemia can be frightening for a patient to experience and may progress to a coma. Care in avoiding hypoglycemia is the priority.
- It is not wise to skip the next dose of insulin when a low glucose level is recorded, especially in patients with type 1 diabetes who do not produce their own insulin; therefore,

will be at risk of diabetic ketoacidosis, which is potentially fatal. Insulin dose may be reduced, but should not be skipped altogether.

- If there is a known reason for high glucose levels (e.g. infection) that requires an insulin dose to be increased temporarily, do not forget to lower the dose again once the problem is resolved.
- Exercising under conditions of near normoglycemia results in increased insulin sensitivity and may necessitate a lowering of insulin dose during the period immediately before as well as immediately after the exercise. Renal impairment decreases insulin clearance and hence doses have to be lowered appropriately. It is important to note that, if a patient is skipping meals, you cannot skip full dose of insulin, instead a small dose has to be still given to act as basal insulin every few hrs or NPH at longer intervals.
- Before making permanent changes in insulin dosage, make sure that high or low blood sugar is not due to unusual diet or exercise. It is desirable to wait for 2 to 3 days before adjusting insulin to correct a high sugar reading unless sugar levels are very high. If the sugar levels are consistently out of range for 2 to 3 days in a row, then adjust the insulin.
- It is recommended that insulin dose be changed by 1 to 2 units at a time. More than 4 units change can be done if the blood sugar values are grossly out of range.

Knowing Which Insulin Component to Adjust based on Blood Sugar Value

- The pre-breakfast short-acting insulin (regular or lispro, or aspart or glulisine) has major action between breakfast and lunch, and its effect is reflected in post breakfast PPBS and prelunch blood sugar levels. It is adjusted based on post-breakfast PPBS and pre-lunch sugar levels.
- The pre lunch short-acting insulin (regular or lispro or aspart or glulisine) has major action between lunch and dinner, and its effect is reflected in post-lunch PPBS and pre-dinner

blood sugar levels. It is adjusted based on post-lunch PPBS and pre-dinner sugar levels.

- The predinner short-acting insulin (regular or lispro or aspart or glulisine) has major action between dinner and bedtime, and its effect is reflected in post-dinner PPBS and bedtime glucose levels. It is adjusted based on post-dinner PPBS and bedtime sugar levels.
- The morning intermediate acting insulin (NPH) has major action between lunch and dinner, and its effect is reflected in post-lunch PPBS and predinner glucose levels. It is adjusted based on post-lunch PPBS and pre-dinner sugar levels.
- The pre-dinner or bedtime intermediate acting NPH insulin has major action overnight, and its effect is reflected in FBS the next morning. It is adjusted based on midnight sugar levels and FBS.
- The effect of all long acting insulins (glargine or detemir or degludec) is reflected in FBS. Hence all long acting insulins are adjusted based on FBS levels.

Glycemic Goals

Below are the target blood glucose levels for nonpregnant adults with diabetes.

A1C	<7.0%
FBS and preprandial blood glucose	80–130 mg/dL (4.4 to 7.2 mmol/L)
Peak postprandial blood glucose	<180 mg/dL (10.0 mmol/L) (80 – 180 is the range)

However, more stringent or less stringent goals may be set based on individual patient factors. In newly diagnosed patients with diabetes, A1C goal can be <6.5%, and in patients with diabetes who are weak with multiple comorbidities, including CVD and advanced renal disease and high hypoglycemic unawareness, A1C goal can be between 7.1% and 8.5%. For palliative care, the aim is to avoid symptomatic hyperglycemia.

Based on the above principles some sample algorithms for adjusting insulin are given below.

Adjusting Insulin Doses in Twice Daily Premix Insulin Regimen

If FBS is greater than 130 mg/dL consistently for 2 to 3 days, increase night NPH insulin. Before making such a change verify that the 3 to 4 am blood glucose is not below 70 mg/dL. If FBS is less than 80 mg/dL, or if there is evidence of hypoglycemia occurring overnight, reduce night NPH insulin by 1 to 2 units (or by 10%)

If blood glucose 2 hours after breakfast is greater than 180 mg/dL, or if blood glucose before lunch is greater than 130 mg/dL, increase morning regular insulin by 1 to 2 units (or more if the sugar level is very high). If blood glucose after breakfast or before lunch is less than 80 mg/dL reduce morning regular insulin by 1 to 2 units (or by 10%)

If blood glucose 2 hours after lunch is consistently greater than 180 mg/dL or if blood glucose before dinner is greater than 130 mg/dL, increase the morning NPH insulin. If blood glucose after lunch or before dinner is less than 80 mg/dL reduce morning NPH insulin by 1 to 2 units (or by 10%)

If blood glucose 2 hours after dinner is greater than 180 mg/dL or if blood glucose at bedtime is greater than 130 mg/dL, increase predinner regular insulin. If blood glucose after dinner or at bedtime is less than 80 mg/dL reduce predinner regular insulin by 1 to 2 units (or by 10%)

Adjusting Insulin Doses in Basal-bolus Regimen (One Dose Long-acting Basal Plus 3-dose Premeal Short-acting Insulin)

If FBS is **greater than 130 mg/dL** for 2 to 3 days in a row, increase basal insulin by 1 to 2 units (or by 10%). Before making such a change, verify that the blood glucose level at around 3 to 4 am is not below 70 mg/dL. **If FBS is less than 80 mg/dL** or if there is evidence of hypoglycemic reactions occurring overnight, reduce basal insulin dose by 1 to 2 units (or by 10%)

If blood glucose 2 hours after breakfast is **greater than 180 mg/dL** or prelunch sugar is **greater than 130 mg/dL**, increase prebreakfast short acting insulin by 1 to 2 units (or 10%). If blood glucose after breakfast or before lunch is **less than 80 mg/dL** or if there is evidence of hypoglycemic reaction between breakfast and lunch, reduce prebreakfast short acting insulin by 1 to 2 units (or by 10%)

Contd...

Contd...

If 2 hours post-lunch PPBS is greater than 180 mg/dL or if predinner blood glucose is greater than 130 mg/dL for 2 to 3 days in a row, increase prelunch short-acting insulin. If blood glucose after lunch or before dinner is less than 80 mg/dL or if there is evidence of hypoglycemic reaction between lunch and dinner, reduce pre lunch short acting insulin by 1 to 2 units
If blood glucose 2 hours after dinner is greater than 180 mg/dL or if blood glucose at bedtime is greater than 130 mg/dL for 2 to 3 days in a row, increase pre dinner short-acting insulin by 1 to 2 units (or 10%). If blood glucose 2 hours after dinner or at bedtime is less than 80 mg/dL or if there is evidence of hypoglycemic reaction between dinner and bedtime, reduce pre dinner short acting insulin by 1 or 2 units (or 10%)

Adjusting Insulin Doses in Patients on Continuous Subcutaneous Insulin Infusion (CSII)

Important Points to Remember

- The basal insulin rate provides continuous basal amounts of insulin. Its effect is primarily reflected in the fasting blood glucose.
- Each pre-meal insulin bolus provides insulin for utilization and storage of food consumed at that meal. The effect of each bolus is reflected in the blood glucose test results after that meal, and (to a lesser extent) before the next meal.

Keeping these points in mind, adjustments are made as follows:

If FBS is greater than 130 mg/dL for 2 to 3 days in a row, increase basal rate of insulin by 1 to 2 insulin units per day or more depending on how high is FBS. Before making such a change, verify that there is no midnight hypoglycemia (not below 70 mg/dL). If FBS is less than 80 mg/dL or if there is evidence of hypoglycemic reactions occurring overnight, reduce the basal insulin by 1 to 2 units
If blood glucose 2 hours after breakfast is greater than 180 mg/dL or if blood glucose before lunch is greater than 130 mg/dL for 2 to 3 days in a row, increase pre breakfast bolus. If blood glucose after breakfast or before lunch is less than 80 mg/dL or if there is evidence of hypoglycemic reaction between breakfast and lunch, reduce pre-breakfast bolus by 1 to 2 insulin units

Contd...

Contd...

If blood glucose 2 hours after lunch is greater than 180 mg/dL or if blood glucose before dinner is greater than 130 mg/dL for 2 to 3 days in a row, increase pre lunch bolus. If blood glucose 2 hours after lunch or before dinner is less than 80 mg/dL or if there is evidence of hypoglycemic reaction between lunch and dinner reduce pre-lunch bolus by 1 to 2 insulin units
If blood glucose 2 hours after dinner is greater than 180 mg/dL or if blood glucose at bedtime is greater than 130 mg/dL for 2 to 3 days in a row, increase pre dinner bolus. If blood glucose after dinner or at bedtime is less than 80 mg/dL or if there is evidence of hypoglycemic reaction between dinner and bedtime, reduce pre-dinner bolus by 1 to 2 insulin units

What to do if 2 hour PPBS after a Meal is High (>180 mg/dL) but Blood Glucose before the Next Meal is Low (<80 mg/dL)

This usually happens with regular insulin because of late peaking, which does not correspond to postprandial rise in blood glucose and fails to control it. Late peaking causes low blood sugar before next meal

It can be avoided by:

1. Changing the timing of premeal short-acting insulin, i.e. give more gap between the injection and meal (e.g. instead of injecting regular insulin 30 min before a meal inject it 45 min to 1 hour before
2. Changing the carbohydrate content of the meal, i.e. eat less carbohydrates and more protein and fat.
3. Changing the site of injection. Inject the insulin into a site of faster absorption
4. Change the short acting insulin; instead of using regular insulin, use one of the fast acting insulin analogues such as lispro or aspart or glulisine, which gets absorbed fast. Peak action of fast acting insulin analogue comes earlier than regular insulin, which will more effectively control postprandial hyperglycemia. In addition, the action of fast acting insulin analogue gets over much earlier and does not reach till next meal which prevents hypoglycemia before the next meal

Insulin Supplements

Supplements are temporary extra insulin doses, used when food or activity pattern is not stable, during intercurrent illness, and to correct unexplained hyperglycemia. These adjustments are made immediately as required. Supplements can be 2 types:

Compensatory supplements: Used to overcome any unanticipated hyperglycemia.

Anticipatory supplements: Given to limit expected hyperglycemia, for example prior to a large meal at a party.

As told earlier supplements are temporary increase in doses of insulin. However, if supplements are required for more than 3 days continuously in a row, then this increased requirement should be incorporated into the basic regimen and continued daily.

Compensatory Insulin Supplements

Used to overcome excessive preprandial hyperglycemia, as well as during periods of acute loss of control, like inter current illness. These are given as outlined below. Patient himself may be taught to adjust the insulin doses, if staying at home.

If FBS or premeal blood sugar is greater than 130 mg per dL, give an extra 1 to 2 insulin units as a supplement at that time **(Table 7.2)**. If FBS or premeal blood sugar is greater than 200 mg per dL, give an extra 2–4 insulin units as a supplement at that time. It is important that the supplement be recorded separately from the basic dose, this helps to prevent inadvertent incorporation of the supplement into the routine daily dose. But if there is a continuing need for a pre-meal supplement indicating consistent hyperglycemia say for 3 days in a row, then this supplemental dose should be incorporated into the daily insulin regimen. It dictates the need for an adjustment of the insulin dose covering the previous meal. For example, if the pre lunch blood sugar is consistently high for 3 days in a row pre lunch supplements should be taken to bring post-lunch glycemia under control, and the pre-breakfast insulin adjusted on the 4th day, which is incorporated into basic regimen and then continued as daily routine dose.

During illness, larger and more frequent supplements may be needed, perhaps as often as every 3–4 hr. Supplements during illness are approximately 1–2 units of insulin for every 30–50 mg per dL that blood glucose exceeds 120 mg/dL.

If glycemic control deteriorates, despite the use of supplements, the magnitude of supplements should be increased (doubled).

Table 7.2: Sample algorithm for use of compensatory insulin supplements based on pre-meal sugar level
<80 mg per dL, reduce the pre-meal dose by 2 units
80 to 130 continue same pre-meal dose
130–150 mg per dL, increase the pre-meal dose by 2 units
150 to 200 mg per dL, increase the pre-meal dose by 3 units
200 to 250 mg per dL, increase the pre-meal dose by 4 units
>250 mg per dL, increase the pre-meal dose by 6 units

Anticipatory Insulin Supplements

This is used to prevent hyperglycemia after a large meal. It is administered before consumption of an anticipated larger than usual meal, e.g. in parties, functions, etc. Start with 1–3 units as an anticipatory supplement for a typical large meal. If the patient has learned carbohydrate counting, insulin can be given proportional to the increment in carbohydrate content of that meal. Tight control of blood glucose requires that the patient participates in the management of their diabetes. This includes monitoring their blood glucose and learning to count carbohydrates or "carb count." The following paragraph explains how to calculate the supplemental dose of short-acting insulin required to cover a meal and how to add extra insulin to correct a hyperglycemic event.

Determining the Dose of Short-acting Insulin to Use before a Meal

Correction for extra large meal; The "Rule of 500"

This is used to determine how many grams of carbohydrate 1 unit of insulin will cover. When this number is known, then the person can easily give the correct dose of insulin by simply counting the grams of carbohydrate they intend to eat at the meal. Specifically, 500 divided by the total daily insulin dose (500/TDI) gives the number of grams of carbohydrate that 1 unit of insulin will cover. For example, if a person has established that they require about 50 units of insulin per day, then it follows that 1 unit of insulin will cover 10 grams of carbohydrate (500/50 = 10). If the person is going to consume extra 100 grams of carbohydrate in the dinner meal, then the extra dose of short acting insulin will be 10 units given before that meal.

Correction for hyperglycemia; the "Rule of 1800"

"Rule of 1800" is used to determine how much insulin to use to bring a high glucose reading back to goal. Even with tight control, hyperglycemia occurs and people need to be able to correct this situation.

Specifically, 1800 divided by the total daily insulin dose yields a value indicating how much 1 unit of insulin will lower the blood glucose. Thus, if a person uses 60 units of insulin per day, then 1 unit of insulin will reduce the blood glucose by 30 mg/dL (1800/60 = 30). Hence, if a person's pre-meal blood glucose is 250 mg/dL, i.e 120 mg more than the expected (expected is less than 130 mg/dL), then we have to give 4 units extra in addition to the usual pre-meal dose of insulin. This extra dose of insulin can be used by itself to correct hyperglycemia which occurs randomly, or added to the bolus dose if glucose is high before a meal.

Adjustments for Exercise

During an unusual activity that is not part of the patient's daily routine, compensation can be made as extra food to provide for increased energy requirements. Initially this may be 10–15 gm carbohydrate for every 30–45 minutes during activity. Blood glucose (by the patient) should be monitored frequently — before, during, and after exercise. Anticipatory insulin decrements may be considered in addition to dietary supplements. Exercise induced hypoglycemia occurs less commonly with CSII. This is because, the exercise induced hypoglycemia is because of rapid absorption of subcutaneous depot insulin, which is not seen in CSII.

Algorithms should be individualized appropriately for the circumstances of any given patient. During pregnancy, one should aim for a FBS of 90 mg/dL and pre lunch, pre dinner and bedtime levels should be ≤105. Anything above this, abovementioned algorithms should be used to control blood sugar.

Sliding Scales

Sliding scales generally refer to giving insulin dose based on pre-meal blood sugar values. The doctor decides how much more insulin supplements should be given along with the usual pre-meal doses when there is high blood sugar levels. Sliding scales are used to adjust short-acting insulins like lispro or regular insulin. They should not be used for the intermediate-acting or long-acting insulins (like NPH or glargine or detemir). In addition to the blood sugar level, expected food intake and exercise following the meal must all be considered to decide the dose of insulin. The blood sugar level Should never be the only factor considered. Illness, stress, and meals etc must also be considered. The dose of short-acting insulin to neutralize a high blood sugar reading may be different for different persons and it should be chosen individually. One advantage of sliding scales is that the blood sugar level must always be measured if the scale is to be used. Sometimes one scale is used for the morning and a different scale for the evening. It may even be necessary to use one scale for an active day and a different scale for a quiet day. It is important to remember that sliding scales are not fixed scales. A scale that works well for a few months may have to be altered if the blood sugars are not in the desired range. The range of insulin is usually preset by the doctor. Patient himself can adjust insulin provided he has good education about diabetes.

Sliding scales are set taking into account all the factors as described earlier. For example, if a person is taking 6 units of short acting insulin before meals, and suppose it has been observed that 1 unit insulin brings down his blood sugar by 25 mg/dL, now if this persons pre-meal blood glucose is 250 mg/dL, he requires his previous usual dose of insulin plus extra 4 units of insulin to cover for his extra 100 mg/dL blood glucose above 150 mg/dL. Hence, his total pre-meal insulin dose would be 10 units. Using this information a sliding scale for this person can be constructed as follows **(Table 7.3)**.

Table 7.3: Sample sliding scale

Pre-meal blood glucose	*Usual insulin dose*	*Extra insulin*	*Total insulin dose*
80 to 150	6	nil	6
150 – 200	6	2	8
200 – 250	6	4	10
250 – 300	6	6	12
>300	6	8	14

(**Note:** If the pre-meal glucose is 155 as above then are you going to give 8 units as per the above table? No, give only six units as 155 is acceptable. And if blood sugar is 175, you can give 7 units. Sliding scales are not foolproof, it is better to err on the safer side than to risk hypoglycemia).

Use of sliding scales is generally discouraged. It is better to use a scheduled dose insulin regimen and use supplemental insulin additionally if required.

Chapter

8

Insulin use during Illness

Illness can disrupt metabolic balance in patients with diabetes. The stress of infection and emotional turmoil is associated with increased release of counter regulatory hormones epinephrine, norepinephrine, glucagon, cortisol and growth hormone. Even relatively mild infections like upper respiratory tract infections or gastrointestinal upset can increase the secretion of counter regulatory hormones. These hormones increase hepatic glucose production, induce a state of insulin resistance with decreased peripheral glucose use, and stimulate ketogenesis. All these factors result in hyperglycemia followed by ketosis. Sometimes acute illness can produce hypoglycemia when these patients receive usual or extra doses of insulin because of diminished food intake, nausea, vomiting and temporary malabsorption.

When a patient is noted to have high blood sugar in the hospital, it may be due to one of the following:

1. *Previously diagnosed diabetes:* This refers to previously diagnosed diabetes whether taking treatment or not. It is already known to patient and treating doctor.
2. *Previously unrecognized diabetes:* Hyperglycemia (FBS ≥126 mg/dL or 2 hours PPBS >200 mg/dL or RBS ≥200 mg/dL or HbA1C ≥6.5%) is noted during hospitalization and confirmed as diabetes after hospitalization by standard diagnostic criteria.
3. *Hospital related hyperglycemia:* Hyperglycemia (FBS ≥126 mg/dL or RBS ≥ 200 mg/dL) is noted during hospitalization and reverts to normal after discharge. But in these patients HbA1C is usually less than 6.5%. This may be due to stress

or iatrogenic due to administration of dextrose containing fluids, glucocorticoids, vasopressors, etc.

Many studies have shown that maintaining normoglycemia during illness improves outcome.

The Cornerstones of Management during Illness Include

- Never stop insulin
- Prevent dehydration and hypoglycemia
- Frequently monitor blood glucose levels
- Monitor for ketosis
- Use supplemental insulin as needed
- Treat the underlying infection or triggering factor
- Review the patient frequently.

Insulin should not be stopped during illness, even if eating is markedly decreased. Insulin requirements may actually go up as explained earlier and supplemental short-acting insulin may have to be given. Supplemental regular insulin may have to be given more frequently say every 3 to 4 hr and if insulin lispro is being used it should be given every 2–3 hr, depending on blood sugar values. If the blood sugar is low, insulin dose has to be decreased.

Hydration should be maintained well. Oral hydration is preferred. The blood sugar level determines whether sugar containing or sugar free fluids should be consumed. When patient is not able to take solid food, and blood glucose is < 180 mg/dL, sugar-containing liquids may be given (juices, soft drinks, etc.) to provide calories. If oral intake is not adequate, additional IV fluids may also be required.

During any intercurrent illness, blood sugars and ketone levels should be monitored every 2–4 hr.

If the patient is on CSII, basal rate should be increased by 20 to 50% during illness, while monitoring blood glucose frequently. Pre-meal boluses should be adjusted to maintain the blood glucose levels in the target range. Always check the infusion site for infection, as this itself may be the site of infection and source of sepsis.

Consider Admission if the Patient has

- An obvious infection requiring parenteral antibiotics
- Illness lasts longer than 2 days
- Vomiting or diarrhea of more than 8 hours
- Blood sugar is over 400 mg in two consecutive tests
- Moderate to large urine or blood ketones with a blood glucose level over 200 mg for more than 8 hours
- Feeling very ill, with extreme fatigue, shortness of breath, or dizziness

Glycemic Targets in Critically Ill Patients

Among hospitalized patients, hyperglycemia, hypoglycemia, and glucose variability are associated with adverse outcomes, including death. Hence good glycemic control is very important in these patients. Many studies suggest that tight glycemic control increases mortality and risk of hypoglycemia compared with more moderate glycemic targets. Hence, for the majority of hospitalized patients ADA recommends a target glucose range of **140–180 mg/dL** for the majority of critically ill and non-critically ill patients. More stringent goals, such as 110–140 mg/dL, may be appropriate for selected patients if they can be achieved without significant hypoglycemia.

Role of Oral Antidiabetic Drugs during Illness

No large-scale studies have investigated the role of oral diabetes agents in hospitalized patients. None of the three primary groups (sulphonylureas, biguanides, and thiazilidinediones) have been studied systematically. Recommendations are largely based on observational studies. The following is the summary of present recommendations regarding use of oral diabetic agents. Each drug should be reviewed in the light of present disease, potential toxicities, and contraindications.

Sodium–glucose cotransporter 2 (SGLT2) inhibitors: SGLT2 inhibitors **should be avoided** in cases of severe illness, in patients with ketonemia or ketonuria, and during prolonged fasting and surgical procedures. SGLT2 inhibitors are not recommended for routine in-hospital use. Furthermore, the

FDA has recently warned that SGLT2 inhibitors should be stopped 3 days before scheduled surgeries (4 days in the case of ertugliflozin).

Glucagon like peptide 1 (GLP-1) receptor agonists and dipeptidyl peptidase 4 inhibitors: These drugs are safe to use in most of the patients. However, consider stopping saxagliptin and alogliptin in patients with heart failure.

Sulphonylureas: There is more propensity for hypoglycemia to occur with these agents in sick patients because of their long duration of action. They do not allow rapid dose adjustment to meet the changing inpatient needs. They should be discontinued in any patient who is nil by mouth (NBM) or unable to take adequate food orally. The pharmacokinetics of sulphonylureas may be altered when there is renal or liver dysfunction. If so, they should be avoided in these situations. Recently the safety of sulphonylureas has been questioned in patients with active coronary artery disease. The phenomenon of ischemic preconditioning has raised concerns about direct effects of sulphonylurea therapy on the myocardium, especially in the setting of acute myocardial injury. KATP channels on beta cells to which sulphonylureas bind are also found in the myocardium. When myocardium is subjected to repeated ischemia before total coronary occlusion myocardium becomes resistant to infarction which is known as ischemic preconditioning. This ischemic preconditioning is dependent on activation of KATP channels which is blocked by sulphonylureas. Studies comparing glimepiride and glibenclamide have shown that glyburide has more of this unwanted side effect. There are no studies on glipizide so far. Hence, it seems reasonable to avoid glibenclamide, at least in patients with active coronary artery disease.

Metformin: Should be withheld the day before any diagnostic evaluation that involves the use of iodinated radio contrast dyes because contrast agents can cause renal damage and it is dangerous to use metformin in the presence of renal failure. It can be restarted 48 hours after radio contrast exposure and documentation of normal renal function. Metformin should be discontinued in the presence of sepsis, CHF, renal dysfunction, or other conditions that predispose to lactic acidosis. Caution should also be used in patients with liver dysfunction, COPD with hypoxia (hypoxia predisposes to lactic acidosis).

Thiazolidinediones (TZDs): Should not be given in the presence of hepatic dysfunction as fatal fulminant liver failure has been documented with the use of these agents. Troglitazone has already been removed from market. Concerns have also been raised about fluid retention caused by these agents, which can worsen heart failure. The initiation of these agents in patients with poorly compensated heart failure is not recommended. It is not wise to use these drugs in acute coronary ischemia in view of possible increase in intravascular volume. Also for inpatient glucose control thiazolidinediones are not suitable because of very slow onset of action, which is mediated through nuclear transcription.

Glucosidase inhibitors: Can be continued unless there is GI disturbance.

In general in a type 2 diabetic patient with mild illness and able to eat normally usual diabetes treatment can be continued, unless specifically contraindicated.

USE OF INSULIN

Insulin when used properly has many advantages in the hospital setting. A key component to provide effective insulin therapy in the hospital setting is to determine whether a patient is insulin deficient or not. Type 1 diabetic patients are by definition insulin deficient. Patient with pancreatectomy or pancreatic dysfunction, history of diabetic ketoacidosis, history of insulin use for more than 5 years, history of diabetes for more than 10 years are likely to have insulin deficiency. All insulin deficient patients must be treated with insulin all the times. In the outpatient setting insulin requirement is divided as basal and prandial needs. Same thing applies to a hospitalized patient if he is eating. However, if the patient is not eating then the insulin needs can be divided as basal and nutritional requirement. Here the nutritional requirement refers to the amount of insulin necessary to cover IV dextrose, TPN, enteral feedings and other nutritional supplements.

An additional factor that may cause increased insulin requirement as explained above is illness related stress. This additional amount of insulin requirement specific to illness is referred to as "illness" or "stress-related insulin" and varies between individuals.

Insulin can be used in many ways in the hospital setting. The following description applies to both type 1 and type 2 diabetes. In a sick diabetes patient blood glucose should be monitored at least 2–4 times a day. Extreme values >300 mg/dL or <60 mg/dL from glucometer reading should be confirmed by lab measurements. Urine or blood ketone bodies should be checked if persistent hyperglycemia is observed in febrile or sick patients. In patients with severe illness, intravenous insulin infusion may be advantageous. Consider discontinuing oral diabetic agents if the patient is not eating.

Determining insulin dose: Check duration of diabetes, weight, dietary habits, previous treatment, the degree of control achieved, presence of any diabetic complications like nephropathy, etc. All this information is crucial in planning insulin therapy. Assessment of compliance with previous insulin therapy is especially important. For example, a patient who reportedly takes a total of 40 units of insulin twice daily at home but is actually not compliant with it can suffer from hypoglycemia attack if this full regimen is instituted on admission. If the patient is already on insulin and is well controlled with that regimen, same may be continued during hospitalization and further adjustments made as necessary. If the patient is not well controlled with previous insulin therapy or is being initiated with insulin for the first time, calculating a weight-based regimen is appropriate. Patients with insulin resistance may require higher doses than calculated from weight.

The usual total daily insulin requirement is 0.3 – 0.6 units/kg/day. Patients who are thin and insulin sensitive may be started with 0.3 units/kg/day, and obese insulin resistant patients may be started at 0.6 units/kg/day. Those with very high insulin resistance may even be started at 1 unit/kg/day. After determining the total daily dose choose one of the following regimens.

Studies have shown that the common practice of sliding scale administration of regular insulin alone 6–8 hourly based on bedside glucometer readings seldom gives satisfactory results especially in insulin deficient individuals like type 1 diabetes and advanced type 2 diabetes. Regimens that include intermediate acting insulin give better glycemic control. Wherever possible provide basal insulin coverage by using intermediate or long acting insulin and prandial coverage by using short-acting insulins.

Insulin use in a Sick Patient Who is able to Take Orally

Any of the following regimens can be used to control blood sugar:

Two-injections daily: For patients who are eating, the estimated total daily insulin is divided into two injections as follows:

- Two-thirds of the total daily dose is administered as premix insulin before breakfast (70% NPH 30% short-acting)
- *One-third of the total daily dose is given as premix before dinner* (50: 50 or OR 70:30 ratio).

Three injections daily: This is also a good option in patients who are taking orally and has more flexibility of timing and dosing than two injections per day.

Option 1

- Short-acting insulin given before breakfast and lunch.
- Premix insulin (70% NPH and 30% short-acting) given before dinner.

Option 2

- Short-acting insulin given before every meal (i.e. before breakfast, lunch, and dinner), a total of three injections per day.
- A small dose of short-acting insulin can also be given before evening snack in addition to mealtime injections which makes it four injections per day.

Four injection per day: There are two options for using a four injection daily regimen for the patient who is able to take orally.

Option 1: Short-acting before each meal and NPH at bedtime (total 4 injections)

- Out of the total dose required, 75% is given as short-acting insulin before each meal (i.e., 25% before breakfast, 25% before lunch, and 25% before dinner. Remaining 25% of the total daily dose is administered at bedtime as NPH insulin.

Option 2: Basal bolus regemen; Short-acting insulin before every meal and long-acting basal insulin at bedtime (total 4 injections)

- Half (50%) of the total daily dose is administered before each meal as ultra short-acting insulin, i.e., 17% before breakfast, 17% before lunch, and 17% before dinner.
- Remaining half (50%) of the total daily dose is administered before bedtime as long acting basal insulin (glargine or detemir or degludec).

Continuous Subcutaneous Insulin Infusion (CSSI)

CSSI provides a continuous basal dose of insulin, combined with as needed bolus doses. It can be continued provided there is adequate supervision by nursing staff. Where this is difficult CSSI should be changed to one of the subcutaneous injection regimens.

Supplemental Insulin Doses

A common misconception is that regular insulin administered 3 or 4 times per day according to sliding scale is sufficient for adequate glycemic control during illness. Insulin given according to sliding scale amounts to corrective action after the blood sugar becomes high, i.e. injections are given when high blood sugar levels are reached. Sliding scale insulin given at mealtimes does not provide overnight coverage and may result in fasting hyperglycemia. Therefore, sliding scale insulin should be used only as a supplemental regimen in conjunction with a scheduled insulin dosage.

Calculation of Supplemental Insulin Dose

Supplemental insulin is administered at meals only. Supplemental insulin use at bedtime or midnight is discouraged because of risk of hypoglycemia. Sliding scale is made by using 5% of the total daily insulin dose as the starting dose. Increments should be of same magnitude. However, note that sliding scales are not rigid scales and can be modified depending on the clinical situation and patient sensitivity to insulin.

Example: If a person is using total 40 units insulin per day, start the sliding scale at 5% of this value, i.e. 2 units and go on adding multiples of 2 units to sliding scale. Hence, for this person sliding scale will be as follows **(Table 8.1)**.

In addition to high blood sugar, if moderate to large ketones are present in the blood or urine, more supplemental insulin may be required. The above sliding scale assumes that the patient's food intake and activity remains consistent. If the pre meal blood sugar is high and if the patient skips that particular meal for any reason then usual dose is skipped and only supplemental insulin administered to avoid hypoglycemia.

Food Intake during Illness

If the patient is too sick to follow usual meal plan, try to replace carbohydrates with liquids or soft foods. Carbohydrates should be provided to prevent fatty acid oxidation and formation of ketone bodies. Carbohydrates also provide the required calories and prevent hypoglycemia. Glycemic effect of carbohydrate depends more on the total amount of carbohydrate rather than the source. Sucrose does not increase blood sugar to a greater extent than isocaloric amounts of starch. Hence the total quantity of carbohydrate is more

Table 8.1: Sample sliding scale

Pre-meal blood sugar level	*Dose of insulin to be given in addition to usual dose as supplement before meals*
70 – 150	Give usual dose
151 – 200	2 units
201 – 250	4 units
251 – 300	6 units
301 – 350	8 units
351 – 400	10 units

important than the type of carbohydrate. Small, frequent feeds are better tolerated during an illness. Advice the patient to take 100–150 ml per hour of sherbheth, fruit juice, ganji, etc. Tea, coffee, etc. can also be taken. Drinking such fluids prevents dehydration and also provides calories. One common mistake is to give sugarless tea, coffee, etc. remember that the body also requires glucose just like it requires insulin. If the patient does not have vomiting, soft foods like, cream soup, cooked cereal, plain yogurt, banana, scrambled egg, custard, etc. can be tried. They should be given in small quantities say half cup at a time. Avoid spicy foods.

Insulin use in a Patient Who is Not able to Take Orally

Patients who are not eating orally still require basal insulin replacement. In addition, these patients may be on enteral feedings, dextrose infusions or other supplements. Hence, these patients require basal insulin replacement given as continuous IV insulin infusion or intermediate acting insulin (NPH) given BD or long acting insulin (glargine or detemir or degludec) given OD. In addition to this, supplemental insulin may be required to cover for enteral feedings, IV dextrose infusions, etc. This additional supplemental insulin may be given as multiple subcutaneous injections (regular insulin 4–6 hr, or insulin lispro or aspart every 4 hours). Some type 2 diabetes patients may have adequate endogenous basal insulin secretion and such patients may achieve good glycemic control with regular insulin only given 4 to 6 times daily subcutaneously. Sometimes glycemic control is achieved with basal insulin replacement itself.

Insulin use in Diabetic Patients on Enteral Feeding (Through Ryle's Tube or Gastrostomy etc.)

During prolonged postoperative recovery, CVA, coma or any other illness, patients may require enteric feeding or TPN (total parenteral nutrition). Enteral feeding may be intermittent or continuous. For intermittent feeding basal insulin may be provided by NPH either once or twice daily. If the patient is being fed only during daytime then give NPH only in the morning. In type 1 diabetics, NPH may have to be given in the night also to provide basal insulin coverage even if the patient is not being fed at night. Regular or lispro or aspart or glulisine insulin can be given before each feed to provide prandial insulin. If the patient is on continuous feeds then NPH may be given twice daily or glargine once daily to provide basal insulin. Additional regular or lispro or aspart insulin can be given subcutaneously as correctional doses (supplements) to correct a high blood sugar reading. Most standard enteric feed formulas contain 12–16% carbohydrate content. Each pack of enteric formula (240 mL) contains 30–40 g carbohydrate. It is usually given at a rate of 100 mL/hour = 12 to 16 gm carbohydrate/hour. Initial insulin dose selection should be based on the previous regimen, degree of stress, and the rate of enteric feeding. Basal insulin requirement would be 1 U/hour and continuous tube feeding at 100 mL/hour (15 g) requires insulin of 2 units per hour. Hence, a total of 3 units/hour of insulin may be required, which is best given as IV infusion. Further adjustments may be made as required.

Insulin use in Diabetic Patients on Total Parenteral Nutrition (TPN)

TPN carbohydrate content is generally 25% dextrose. Therefore, most diabetics will require insulin cover during TPN. Insulin infusion is the best method for management. Though insulin can be added into the TPN bag, a separate line for IV insulin infusion offers more flexibility of dose adjustment. Many type 2 diabetic patients may require up to 100 units or more of insulin per day to achieve blood sugar control.

Intravenous Insulin Infusion

IV insulin is used in DKA, HHS. Any critically ill patient with unacceptable hyperglycemia for 24 – 48 hours is a candidate for IV insulin infusion especially if it is not responding to increasing doses of subcutaneous regimen. Regular insulin or lispro insulin is used for IV infusion. There is no advantage of lispro or aspart over regular insulin when used as intravenous infusion. Blood glucose should be monitored every 1–2 hourly when using IV infusion. While discontinuing insulin infusion and changing over to subcutaneous regimen, the first dose of SC injection should be given one hour before discontinuing IV infusion. This is because half-life of IV insulin is only 5 min and discontinuing it before overlapping with SC insulin results in rapid dissipation of insulin levels which may result in hyperglycemia. Type 1 DM patients without endogenous insulin secretory capacity are more prone to this. An insulin infusion protocol known as Yale insulin infusion protocol (developed by Yale New Haven Hospital) for use in critically ill patients is given in **Table 8.2**. Note that this infusion protocol does not apply to DKA and HHS.

Yale Insulin Infusion Protocol

The following insulin infusion protocol is intended for use in hyperglycemic adult patients in an ICU setting, but is not specifically tailored for those individuals with diabetic emergencies, such as diabetic ketoacidosis (DKA) or hyperglycemic hyperosmolar states (HHS). When these diognoses are being considered or if BG ≥500 mg/dL, an MD should be consulted for specific orders. Also, please notify an MD if the response to the insulin infusion is unusual or unexpected, or if any situation arises that is not adequately addressed by these guidelines.

Initiating an Insulin Infusion

1. Insulin infusion: Mix 1 U regular human insulin per 1 cc 0.9% NaCl. Administer via infusion pump (in increments of 0.5 U/hr)
2. Priming: Flush 50 cc of indusion through all IV tubing before infusion begins (to saturate the insulin binding sites in the tubing)
3. Target blood glucose (BG) levels: 100–139 mg/dL
4. Bolus and initial insulin infusion rate: Divide initial BG level by 100, then round to nearest 0.5 U for bolus and initial infusion rate

Examples:
1. Initial BG = 325 mg/dL: 325 + 100 = 3.25, round ↑ to 3.5: IV bolus 3.5 U + start infusion @ 3.5 U/hr
2. Initial BG = 174 mg/dL: 174 + 100 = 1.74, round ↓ to 1.5: IV bolus 1.5 U + start infusion @ 1.5 U/hr

Blood Glucose (BG) Monitoring

1. Check BG hourly until stable (3 consecutive values within target range). In hypotensive patients, capillary blood glucose (i.e., fingersticks) may be inaccurate and obtaining the blood sample from an indwelling vascular catheter is acceptable.

Contd...

Contd...

2. Then check BG q 2 hours; once stable × 12–24 hours. BG checks can be spaced to q 4 hours IF:
   a. No significant change in clinical condition and
   b. No significant change in nutritional intake.
3. If any of the following occur, consider the temporary resumption of hourly BG monitoring, until BG is again stable (2–3 consecutive BG values within target range):
   a. Any change in insulin infusion rate (i.e., BG out of target range)
   b. Significant changes in clinical condition
   c. Initiation or cessation of pressor or steroid therapy
   d. Initiation or cessation of renal replacement therapy (hemodialysis, CVVH, etc.)
   e. Initiation, cessation, or rate change of nutritional support (TPN, PPN, tube feedings, etc.)

	Changing the Insulin Infusion Rate		
If BG <50 mg/dL: D/C insulin infusion	Give 1 amp (25 g) D 50 IV: Recheck BG q 15 minutes. ➔When BG ≥100 mg/dL, wait 1 hour, then restart insulin infusion at 50% original rate		
If BG 50–74 mg/dL: D/C insulin infusion	If symptomatic (or unable to assess), give 1 amp (25 g) D50 IV; recheck BG q 15 minutes. If asymptomatic,1/2 amp (12.5 g) D50 IV or 8 ounces juice; recheck BG q 15–30 minutes ➔When BG ≥ 100 mg/dL, wait 1 hour, then restart infusion at 75% original rate		
If BG ≥ 75 mg/dL:			
Step 1: Determine the current BG Level – identifies a column in the table:			
BG 75–99 mg/dL	***BG 100–139 mg/dL***	***BG 140–199 mg/dL***	***BG ≥200 mg/dL***

Step 2: Determine the Rate of Change from the prior BG level—identifies a CELL in the table – Then move right for Instructions:

[**Note:** If the last BG was measured 2–4 hr before the current BG, calculate the hourly rate of change. Example: If the BG at 2 pm was 150 mg/dL and the BG at 4 pm is now 120 mg/dL, the total chagne over 2 hours is – 30 mg/dL; however, the hourly change is – 30 mg/dL ÷ 2 hours = – 15 mg/dL/hour]

Contd...

Contd...

BG 75–99 mg/dL	***BG 100–139 mg/dL***	***BG 140–199 mg/dL***	***BG ≥200 mg/dL***	***Instructions****
		BG ↑ by > 50 mg/dL/hr	BG ↑	↑ Infusion by "2Δ"
	BG ↑ by > 25 mg/dL/hr	BG ↑ by 1–50 mg/dL/hr OR BG Unchanged	BG Unchanged OR BG ↓ by 1–25 mg/dL/hr	↑ Infusion by "Δ"
BG ↑	BG ↑ by 1–25 mg/dL/hr BG Unchanged OR BG ↓ by 1–25 mg/dL/hr	BG ↓ by 1–50 mg/dL/hr	BG ↓ by 26–75 mg/dL/hr	No Infusion Change
BG Unchanged OR BG ↓ by 1–25 mg/dL/hr	BG ↓ by 26–50 mg/dL/hr	BG ↓ by 51–75 mg/dL/hr	BG ↓ by 76–100 mg/dL/hr	Decrease Infusion by "Δ"
BG ↓ by >25 mg/dL/hr *see below*	BG ↓ by >50 mg/dL/hr	BG ↓ by >75 mg/dL/hr	BG ↓ by >100 mg/dL/hr	Hold × 30 min, then ↓ infusion by "2Δ"
D/C Insulin Infusion; BG q 30 min; when BG ≥ 100 mg/dL, restart infusion @75 % of most recent rate				

***Changes in Infusion Rate ("Δ") are determined by the current rate:**		
Current Rate (U/hr)	***Δ = Rate change (U/hr)***	***2Δ = 2X Rate change (U/hr)***
< 3.0	0.5	1
3.0–6.0	1	2
6.5–9.5	1.5	3
10–14.5	2	4
15–19.5	3	6
20–24.5	4	8
≥25	≥5	10 (consult MD)

Fig. 8.1: Yale insulin infusion protocol. [Copyright © 2004 American Diabetes Association. From Diabetes Care, Vol. 27, 2004; 461-467. Reprinted with permission from The American Diabetes Association]

YALE INSULIN INFUSION PROTOCOL

Yale insulin infusion protocol has been tested in critically ill patients and is very effective in controlling blood sugars. It takes into account current blood glucose levels and infusion rate as well as hourly rate of change of blood sugars to determine the infusion rate. The median time to reach target blood glucose levels (100–139 mg/dL) was 9 hours by using Yale insulin infusion protocol. Only 0.3% of the blood glucose values were in the hypoglycemic range (<60 mg/dL).

Planning Discharge

Most patients can be returned to their previous diabetic regimen of either insulin or OHAs. If possible, the final outpatient regimen should be initiated at least 24 hours in advance of discharge. As the patient comes back to his usual life further adjustments may be required after discharge. Hence, follow up care is also important. Patient should be educated about hypoglycemia symptoms and methods to correct it. Patients with no prior history of diabetes who are found to have hyperglycemia during hospitalization are likely to be diagnosed as diabetes at follow up testing (up to 60% may be diagnosed as diabetes). Hence, such patients should be retested within 1 month of discharge for diabetes.

Chapter

9

Perioperative Management of Diabetes

Any surgery is a stress even for normal people. The morbidity and mortality rates during the perioperative period are more in diabetics than in non-diabetics. More number of surgeries are also done in diabetics than non-diabetics (like ophthalmological procedures, cardiovascular surgeries and limb amputations, which are more common in diabetics). Many diabetics have impaired renal function and are prone to fluid and electrolyte imbalances.

A diabetic is more prone for the following:

- Fluid and electrolyte imbalances, dehydration.
- Higher incidence of wound infection, UTI, pneumonia, and other systemic infections. Infections account for two-thirds of all postoperative complications and 20% of all postoperative deaths.
- Delayed wound healing and as a consequence, increased incidence of wound dehiscence. This is because collagen synthesis is suppressed by hyperglycemia higher than 200 mg/dL. Granulocyte chemotaxis and phagocytic action is also affected by hyperglycemia especially when >250 mg/dL.

METABOLIC CHANGES IN A DIABETIC DURING SURGERY

Many metabolic changes occur during surgery that have an effect on diabetes. The stress of anesthesia and surgery increases the secretion of epinephrine, norepinephrine, cortisol and growth hormone which are all insulin antagonists and cause insulin resistance at tissue level. Epinephrine also suppresses insulin secretion. There is increase in gluconeogenesis. There is also increased catabolism of proteins during and after surgery. All these factors contribute to hyperglycemia during and after surgery. Uncontrolled hyperglycemia instigates osmotic diuresis (causing fluid and electrolyte imbalance), ketogenesis, and increased generation of pro-inflammatory cytokines with resultant mitochondrial injury, endothelial dysfunction, and immune deregulation. Hence, achieving good glucose control during the perioperative period is associated with beneficial post-surgical outcomes.

The extent of the metabolic changes depend on the type of surgery, the length of surgery, the stress of surgery and the type of anaesthesia used. Increased glucose elevation is seen more commonly in cases of general anesthesia or thoracic/ abdominal surgeries as opposed to epidural/local anesthesia or peripheral/laparoscopic surgeries. Whether the surgery is elective or emergency also affects the extent of metabolic changes. The type of diabetes (whether types 1 or 2), extent of preoperative diabetic control also affects the glycemic control during perioperative period.

Diabetic patients are also at risk of hypoglycemia in the perioperative period. Factors which contribute to perioperative hypoglycemia include prolonged fasting, medications, inadequate nutrition, sedation, and postoperative gastrointestinal problems (vomiting, ileus, gastroparesis, etc).

The perioperative period is divided into three phases:
- Preoperative
- Intraoperative
- Postoperative

Preoperative Assessment

Should include evaluation for any cardiovascular, neurological, or other medical disorder. The status of diabetes, duration, medications, etc. should be assessed. It is also important to know about the type of surgery, time of surgery and the route of anesthesia, as all these will affect glucose control. All patients should have their electrolytes and renal function tests checked. ECG should be done for all. Additional tests may be ordered if necessary. In general, the following assessment should be done in all patients.

Identify Diabetes Type

- Type 1 diabetes indicates absolute need for insulin therapy and requires both basal insulin and prandial insulin (short or rapid acting insulin).
- Type 2 diabetes is associated with increased insulin needs during surgery.

Determine level of preceding glycemic control:

- Review blood glucose records
- Review glycosylated hemoglobin values

Determine presence of diabetic complications:

- Nephropathy (important implications regarding fluid balance, drug dosages)
- Neuropathy (autonomic—arrhythmias, postural hypotension, gastroparesis, bladder dysfunction — urinary retention)

Assess cardiovascular system:

- Coronary artery disease
- Hypertension
- Congestive heart failure

Oral medications and non-insulin injectable agents (GLP-1 analogues) during perioperative period

It is better not to use any oral antidiabetic agents during perioperative period. Metformin can lead to the development of lactic acidosis in cases of renal dysfunction or with the use of intravenous contrast. Sulfonylureas and other insulin secretagogues may lead to hypoglycemia. Sodium-glucose cotransporter-2 (SGLT-2) inhibitors carry the risk of volume depletion due to osmotic dieresis and euglycemic ketoacidosis in fasting, or acutely ill patients. Glucagon-like-peptide-1 receptor (GLP-1) agonists can worsen nausea and vomiting by delaying gastric emptying. Delayed onset and long duration of action make it difficult to adjust these medicines to achieve optimal glycemic control over a short period. Even though some studies have shown that DPP-4 inhibitors are safe in medical and surgical patients with mild to moderate hyperglycemia, ADA (American Diabetes Association), does not recommend the use of DPP-4 inhibitors in the inpatient setting. Moreover, saxagliptin (a DPP-4 inhibitor) predisposes to heart failure.

Hence, all oral agents should be withheld on the day of surgery. SGLT-2 inhibitors should be withheld much before surgery, i.e. 24 to 48 hours before surgery. In cases of emergency surgery or illness, stop all oral agents immediately.

Glycemic Targets during Perioperative Period

Aim for a target blood glucose levels of 80 – 180 mg/dL. Glycemic control tighter than 80–180 mg/dL does not improve outcomes and is associated with more hypoglycemia. Management plans are given below, depending on the above factors.

Management of Diabetes during Perioperative Period

Patients undergoing minor surgery (e.g. cystoscopy, incision and drainage) whose diabetes is controlled with diet or oral medicines do not need insulin during surgery.

For all other types of surgeries, it is ideal to start on insulin. Skip all the oral agents on the day of surgery and immediate postoperative period. These oral medicines may be restarted, when the patient resumes his usual diet.

There are two ways of managing diabetes during perioperative period, either by using subcutaneous insulin injections or by using intravenous insulin infusion.

Subcutaneous Insulin Injections

Most of the patients with diabetes can be managed with subcutaneous insulin perioperatively. Patients who are on insulin should be instructed to continue their usual meal plan and insulin regimen until the night before surgery. Give the usual dose of long-acting insulin on the night before surgery; however, if the patient reports a history of nocturnal or fasting hypoglycemia, reduce the basal insulin dose by 20 to 25%. If the patient is taking the basal insulin in the morning daily, then give the morning dose on the day of surgery but reduce the dose by 20–25%. Remember that basal insulin is mandatory and should not be skipped entirely.

Skip the prandial short or rapid acting insulin when the patient is fasting and kept NBM.

If the patient is taking premixed insulin combinations (70/30, 75/25, 50/50), give the usual evening dose of premix insulin the night prior to surgery, but skip the morning dose of premix insulin on the day of surgery. But NPH component of premix insulin can be given in the morning of surgery at a reduced dose (reduce by 25 to 50%) to provide basal coverage. Another option is to discontinue the patient's premixed insulin and change to a regimen involving long-acting insulin (i.e. glargine) to be administered the night before surgery.

Hyperglycemia can be corrected with short-acting or rapid-acting insulin based on the patient's insulin sensitivity: regular insulin is given every 6 hours or rapid-acting insulin (aspart, lispro, or glulisine) every 4 hours.

Intravenous Continuous Insulin Infusion

The major disadvantage of multiple subcutaneous injections given subcutaneously is the variable and unpredictable insulin absorption. Because of this, extremes of blood glucose levels frequently occur (either hyper- or hypoglycemia). Once administered, the insulin effect cannot be modified and if the operation is delayed by a few hours, patient may develop hypoglycemia. Use of sliding scales based on blood glucose values (or worse urine glucose values), to correct hyperglycemia results in retrospective care and causes roller coaster like blood glucose levels. Therefore, regimens consisting of continuous infusion of regular or lispro insulin are widely used to control hyperglycemia during perioperative period. Continuous intravenous insulin infusion is the most rational and physiological method for perioperative management which has been shown to be safe, effective and flexible by many studies.

Critically ill patients, insulin-treated patients undergoing longer and complicated surgeries or patients with labile type 1 diabetes should always be managed with an intravenous insulin infusion. Blood glucose should be monitored at least hourly and infusion rate should be adjusted accordingly. Aim for a target blood glucose levels of 80–180 mg/dL.

Estimating Insulin Infusion Rate

There is no absolute method for correctly predicting insulin needs in surgical patients. Most surgical patients can be maintained in the 80–180 mg/dL blood glucose range with an insulin infusion 1–2 units/hour. However, many other factors, like type of diabetes, previous therapy, degree of glycemic control, obesity, renal failure, infection, steroid therapy, etc. should be taken into account. Steroid therapy in patients undergoing kidney transplantation will cause twofold to threefold increase in insulin needs. Patients undergoing CABG surgery may require threefold to fivefold increase in insulin, because of use of sympathomimetic drugs, induction of hypothermia and use of glucose-enriched solutions for pump priming. For details given in **Table 9.1**.

Insulin infusion should be started in the morning of surgery, preferably at about the same time that the morning injection is usually administered. For early morning procedures and those needing improved glycemic control, infusion should

Table 9.1: Estimation of insulin infusion rate in surgical patients
For insulin treated diabetics (both type 1 and type 2) with >50 U/day, selected regular insulin dose is 36 U/day
Administered as 1.5 U/hour (36 U/day)
For patients treated with diet, oral agents, or insulin <50 U/day, selected regular insulin dose is 24 U/day
Administered as 1 U/hour (24 U/day) with further adjustments as required
Further dose modifications can be made as follows: ***Conditions associated with increased insulin needs :*** • Previous poor BG control (average FBS >240 mg/dL, HbA1C >10%), selected dose x 1.5 • Obesity, hepatic disease, selected dose x1.5 • Severe infection, steroid therapy, selected dose x 2
Type of surgery: • General surgery: Use selected dose • Renal transplant: Selected dose × 2 • Coronary artery bypass graft, selected dose × 3 – 5 *[**Note:** Regular insulin infusion rate (U/hour) = dose ÷ 24.]*

be started in the night before surgery. However, if this is not possible, start the infusion at least 2–3 hours before surgery. Allowing more time between the start of insulin infusion and surgery will allow more time for titration to the desired level of control. For those using CSII (continuous subcutaneous insulin infusion), it is not critical to start insulin infusion early in the morning as these patients continue to receive basal insulin.

Bedside monitoring should be done every 1–2 hours and if the facilities are not available for this, it is not safe to start insulin infusion. During surgery, anesthesiologist should monitor blood glucose every hour and adjust the infusion of insulin accordingly (if necessary a close liaison with a physician should be maintained through phone). Glucometers are enough to monitor blood glucose. But if the patient is hemodynamically or metabolically unstable, then lab blood glucose measurements should be used, as capillary blood glucose measurements in such patients is unreliable.

Both insulin and glucose infusion are needed during perioperative period. There are 2 ways of doing this. The preferred method is separate infusion of insulin and separate infusion of glucose (5% DNS, 5% dextrose, 5% dextrose in ½ saline). The main advantage of this is that insulin infusion and glucose infusion can be adjusted independently. Dextrose containing fluid is given at the rate of 100 ml/hour in a diabetic patient unless there are contraindications for this such as heart failure, renal failure, etc. where the rate of infusion may have to be reduced. NS is not advised as patients may develop hypoglycemia, severe catabolism and inadequate calories to meet basal energy need.

Increased insulin may be needed in obesity (2–3 U/hour), sepsis (3–4 U/hour), steroid therapy (3 to 4 U/hour), and coronary artery bypass surgery (4–6 U/hour).

The goal should be to maintain a blood glucose level of 80–180 mg/dL. Physicians should be careful when temporarily stopping the insulin infusion. Stopping insulin even for short periods may cause rapid dissipation of insulin action and rapid deterioration of metabolic control. This is because the plasma half-life of intravenous insulin is only 5 minutes.

Separate Insulin and Dextrose Infusion during Surgery

This is the preferred method of insulin infusion during perioperative period **(Table 9.2)**. Separate infusion of insulin and separate infusion of glucose (5% DNS, 5% dextrose, 5% dextrose

Table 9.2: Starting separate insulin and dextrose infusion during surgery

- Mix 50 units of regular insulin (human) in 50 mL normal saline (1 U / mL)
- Flush 3 – 5 mL of this fluid through IV line before connecting to patient (because insulin binds to IV tubing and flushing it helps in saturating the binding sites). Connect insulin line to the perioperative fluid maintenance line.
- Perioperative maintenance fluid: Fluids must contain 5% dextrose. Give at the rate of 100 mL/hour unless there is some contraindication like renal failure, CCF, etc.
- Monitor blood glucose (BG) hourly, intraoperatively and postoperatively
- Adjust insulin drip rate as below based on blood glucose values.

BG (mg/dL)	*Insulin infusion rate (Units/hour)*
<80	0.0
81–100	0.5
101–140	1.0
141–180	1.5
181–220	2.0
221–260	2.5
261–300	3.0
301–340	4.0
>341	5.0

- If anytime BG <80 mg/dL, stop insulin and administer intravenous bolus of 50% dextrose (25 mL) and wait for 30 minutes. Once BG >80, restart insulin infusion at 70% of the previous infusion rate. It may be necessary to modify the algorithm
- **You can also put 50 units of insulin in 500 ml NS, i.e. 1 unit = 10 mL. This may be easier to use in infusion pump.** [Note: Blood glucose value ÷ 100 gives a reasonable estimate of infusion dosage (U/hour). For example, if blood sugar value is 500, 500 ÷ 100 = 5, start infusion at 5 units per hour and modify depending on blood sugar measurements. Also see Yale insulin infusion protocol]

in ½ saline) are started. The main advantage of this is that insulin infusion and glucose infusion can be adjusted independently.

Combined Insulin and Dextrose Infusion

This is a less flexible method poorly suited to lengthy and complicated surgical procedures (especially renal transplant and CABG). It is generally not adequate for type 1 diabetics who are prone for wide swings in blood glucose levels. It may be acceptable for elective procedures in type 2 diabetic patients, during which insulin requirements may not vary much. If a patient requires extra insulin while being treated with combined insulin, it may be administered subcutaneously **(Table 9.3)**.

Perioperative management of patients on continuous subcutaneous insulin infusion

Data are limited on use of CSII in the perioperative period, but some reports suggest that it is safe for use during minor

Table 9.3: Starting combined insulin and dextrose infusion during surgery
Patients treated with diet, oral agents, or insulin <50 U/day
• BG <120 mg/dL: Add 5 units of insulin to 1000 mL of 5% dextrose plus 20 mEq KCl
• BG = 120 – 180 mg/dL: Add 10 U insulin
• Blood glucose (BG) > 180 mg/dL: add 15 units of insulin
• Check BG hourly
• Infuse at 100 mL/hour (1 U/hour)
Patients treated with insulin >50 U/day
• BG <120 mg/dL: Add 10 units of insulin to 1000 mL of 5% dextrose plus 20 mEq KCl
• BG = 120 – 180 mg/dL: Add 15 U insulin
• BG >180 mg/dL: Add 20 units of insulin
• Check BG hourly
• Infuse at 100 mL/hour
If BG <80 mg/dL: Stop infusion and administer 25 mL of 50% dextrose IV. Once BG >80, restart insulin infusion. Insulin needs are more for obesity, sepsis, steroid therapy, renal transplant, and coronary artery bypass

procedures. For minor procedures lasting less than 2 hours or same day procedures, it is generally acceptable for patients to continue on their pump by maintaining their outpatient basal rate.

For major or longer surgical procedures, the decision of whether to continue insulin pump management during surgery is usually made on an individual basis. This decision should be made based on patients and hospital staff's ability to manage insulin pump. Alternatively patients managed on insulin pumps should be converted to an intravenous insulin infusion on admission.

Postoperative Period

Insulin infusion should be continued until the patient starts taking orally, and then subcutaneous injections may be started. Continue insulin infusion for 1 to 2 hours after giving the initial subcutaneous dose of regular insulin before stopping infusion. During the reintroduction of foods such as clear liquids, it is preferable to continue a low maintenance insulin infusion supplemented with small doses of subcutaneous regular insulin. The supplement dose depends on the carbohydrate content of the food (Approx 1 unit for 10 gm).

Once the patient can eat adequately, a previously insulin treated diabetic may be started on usual dose or dose based on previous 24 to 48 hour insulin requirements. The dose selected should be 80 to 100% of the previous day's total dose. Requirements may be higher during persistent stress, infection, pain, steroids, or high food intake (total parenteral nutrition).

Patients who were not on insulin before admission for surgery may require insulin postoperatively for some time or few days. In such patients, a subcutaneous regimen totaling 0.2 to 0.5 units/kg of body weight depending on the patient's insulin sensitivity is selected. The selected total daily insulin dose is then divided into a 50% basal component (long-acting insulin) and 50% prandial boluses (rapid-acting insulin) split between breakfast, lunch, and dinner. In addition to scheduled subcutaneous insulin, we can add supplemental doses of insulin as correction to mealtime insulin to correct any unexpected glucose excursions using a sliding scale. Prolonged use of sliding scale is not recommended as the sole treatment as this regimen only passively reacts to hyperglycemia but does not abrogate its development.

Some postoperative patients may require enteral or parenteral nutrition. It is important to monitor blood glucose levels even in previously normoglycemic patients as enteral/parenteral is known to cause hyperglycemia. For enteral feeds, it is recommended to administer basal insulin and use a correctional sliding scale. For parenteral feeds, insulin should be added to the total parenteral nutrition bag and additional correctional insulin administered as needed. If feeds are abruptly discontinued, remember to start a dextrose-containing infusion to avoid potential risk of hypoglycemia. Hypoglycemia may be detected on blood glucose testing.

After discharge, a follow-up visit within one month of discharge is advisable for all patients. An earlier appointment within 1 to 2 weeks is preferred if there has been a change in medications, or glycemic control is not optimal at the time of discharge.

Chapter

10

Insulin use in Pregnancy

Before the discovery of insulin in 1922, most young diabetic women died before the childbearing age and in those who reached childbearing age, there was greater than 90% infant mortality rate and 30% maternal mortality rate. With the discovery of insulin and improved management strategies, the mortality rates have now come down approximately to the same level seen in general population.

When high blood sugars are noted in a pregnant woman, try to categorize what type of diabetes she may be having. Patients with type 1 diabetes are typically diagnosed during an episode of hyperglycemia, ketosis, and dehydration; this occurs most commonly in childhood or adolescence before pregnancy. However, rarely some type 1 diabetes patients may present for the first time during pregnancy and may present as unexpected coma because early pregnancy may provoke diet and glycemic control instability. A pregnancy test should be ordered in all reproductive-aged women admitted to the hospital for blood sugar management. Differentiating type 2 diabetes mellitus from gestational diabetes is very difficult during pregnancy because severe forms of GDM have similar clinical characteristics. Some women who are diagnosed to have GDM in early pregnancy may be found to have overt diabetes after delivery. Although a first-trimester HbA1C value of 8% or more is highly suggestive of pre-existing type 2 diabetes, definitive diagnosis of type 2 diabetes must be made after pregnancy using the 75 g, 2 hour glucose tolerance test. However, whatever may be the type of diabetes during pregnancy, treatment essentially remains the same.

METABOLIC CHANGES DURING PREGNANCY

In a normal non-diabetic woman, glucose level is maintained within a narrow range. In fact, glucose levels are actually lower in pregnant women than in non-pregnant women. This is because the fetus continuously uses maternal blood glucose. Another change is that plasma ketone levels are several times higher, and free fatty acids are elevated after an overnight fast. This is because the body tries to make use of alternative sources of fuel while sparing glucose for fetus. Glucose is transported to the fetus by facilitated diffusion.

The hormonal changes occurring in pregnancy will affect the glucose homeostasis. These include rise in the levels of human placental lactogen (HPL), estrogen, progesterone, cortisol, etc. HPL has the strongest insulin antagonistic action. Although the maternal blood glucose levels remain below non-pregnant levels, insulin levels increase markedly because of the antagonistic action of all these hormones causing insulin resistance. There is also increased degradation of insulin by placental enzymes, which is compensated by increased secretion from pancreas. The increased need for insulin during pregnancy, may cause worsening of diabetes or unmask previously latent diabetes, which results in gestational diabetes.

If the mother has hyperglycemia, fetus also will be exposed to continuous or intermittent hyperglycemia, which in turn increases fetal insulin secretion. Fetal hyperglycemia with high insulin levels may cause malformations (macrosomia), low potassium (and hence predispose to cardiac arrhythmias), inhibition of pulmonary surfactant synthesis (predisposing to respiratory distress of the newborn). Neonatal hypoglycemia due to excess insulin may cause permanent neurologic damage. Maternal hyperglycemia may lead to polyhydramnios, hypertension, UTI, candida vaginitis, abortions, and infertility. All these complications will increase infant and maternal mortality as explained earlier. The infant mortality is directly related to maternal hyperglycemia.

In addition, diabetes in pregnancy may increase the risk of obesity, hypertension, and type 2 diabetes in offspring later in life.

Diagnosis of Gestational Diabetes

The definition of gestational diabetes mellitus (GDM) is any degree of glucose intolerance with onset or first recognition during pregnancy. This definition helps for diagnosis of unrecognized pre-existing diabetes also.

All women who are planning for pregnancy with risk factors for diabetes (obesity, family history) should be screened for undiagnosed diabetes. All pregnant women should be screened for diabetes as early as possible at the first trimester itself.

Testing for GDM is recommended twice during ANC (antenatal care). The first testing should be done during first antenatal visit as early as possible in pregnancy. The second testing should be done during 24–28 weeks of pregnancy if the first test is negative. It is important to ensure second test as many pregnant women develop blood sugar intolerance during this period (24–28 weeks). Moreover, only one-third of GDM positive women are detected during first trimester. If it could not be done during this time, then it can be done any time after 24 weeks of pregnancy. There should be at least 4 weeks gap between the two tests.

The test is to be conducted for all pregnant women even if she comes late in pregnancy for ANC at the time of first contact. If she presents beyond 28 weeks of pregnancy, only one test is to be done at the first point of contact.

Test to Diagnose GDM — 75 gm OGTT

There is no international consensus regarding timing of screening method and the optimal cut-off points for diagnosis and intervention of GDM. Inconsistencies in the GDM diagnostic criteria between different guidelines have led to challenges in making clinical diagnosis. Some organizations do not recommend measuring 1 hour plasma glucose. Most of the organizations recommend 75 gm oral glucose tolerance test (OGTT). In spite of all these inconsistencies, the recommendation by IADPSG (International Association of the Diabetes and Pregnancy Study Groups) criteria have been adopted internationally. IADPSG recommends single step testing using 75 gm oral glucose and blood sugar is measured at 1 and 2 hours after ingestion.

75 gm glucose is to be given orally after dissolving in approximately 300 ml in a fasting state. The intake of the solution has to be completed within 5–10 minutes. Blood sugar is measured at 1 and 2 hours after the oral glucose load. If vomiting occurs within 30 minutes of oral glucose intake, the test has to be repeated the next day. If vomiting occurs after 30 minutes, the test continues.

The diagnosis of GDM is made when any of the following plasma glucose values are met or exceeded following 75 gm OGTT:

- Fasting: 92 mg/dL
- 1 h: 180 mg/dL
- 2 h: 153 mg/dL

Diagnostic criteria for GDM recommended by different organizations are given in **Table 10.1**.

Table 10.1: Diagnostic criteria for GDM recommended by different organizations

Guidelines	*OGTT*	*Fasting PG Mg/dL*	*1-hour PG Mg/dL*	*2-hour PG Mg/dL*	*3-hour PG Mg/dL*
WHO 2013	75 g	92 – 125	Not required	≥140	Not required
ACOG	100 g	≥95	≥180	≥155	≥140
Canadian Diabetes Association	75 g	≥95	≥191	≥160	Not required
IADPSG	75 g	≥92	≥180	≥153	Not required
DIPSI	75 g	Not required	Not required	≥140	Not required

MANAGEMENT

Glucose targets vary among countries and the precise target for optimum maternal, fetal, and newborn outcome is not well-established. The following upper limits are recommended by American Diabetes Association (ADA) and the American College of Obstetricians and Gynecologists (ACOG). If these upper limits are exceeded, then treatment in the form of medical nutrition therapy, oral drugs, or insulin therapy are required.

- FBS: <95 mg/dL
- PPBS: either 1-h postprandial glucose <140 mg/dL or 2-h postprandial glucose <120 mg/dL
- A1C <6% if this can be achieved without significant hypoglycemia, but may be relaxed to <7% if necessary to prevent hypoglycemia.

Medical Nutrition Therapy

All women with GDM should receive nutritional counseling and nutrition therapy. However, it should meet the caloric and nutrient needs of pregnancy and should be tried when FBS <105 mg/dL. Approximately 30–40 kcal/kg ideal body weight or an additional 300 kcal/day above the basal requirement is needed. Total calories should be distributed wisely throughout the day. Breakfast can be split into two equal halves and consumed with a two-hour gap in between. By this, the undue peak in plasma glucose level after breakfast is avoided (note that peaking of blood sugar is high with breakfast than with lunch and dinner due to Dawn phenomenon). For example, if four idlis are consumed for breakfast at 8 am the same can be eaten as two at 8 am and two at 10 am. This will reduce the post breakfast peak in plasma glucose by 20–30 mg/dL. The aim of nutritional therapy is to achieve the following glucose levels. FPG <95 mg/dL, or 1-hour PPG <120 mg/dL. When nutritional therapy fails to maintain glucose at the above levels insulin should be used.

Pharmacologic Therapy

If the glucose targets cannot be maintained by medical nutrition therapy, then pharmacotherapy in the form of oral drugs or insulin should be initiated. Only two oral drugs (metformin and glibenclamide also known as gyburide) are used in pregnancy. In general, insulin is the preferred therapy compared to oral drugs, because it is more effective, easily adjustable, and safe for the fetus, whereas data are lacking regarding long-term outcomes of offspring exposed to oral drugs. However, in those who are not willing for frequent follow ups and donot comply with insulin injections, oral drugs are reasonable alternatives.

Oral Drugs

Only two drugs, metformin and glibenclamide (known as glyburide in many countries) are used in pregnancy as data is not available with other drugs. Both drugs cross the placenta, and no one drug is superior to other drug. Metformin is usually started at the dose of 500 mg orally once daily (with dinner). The dose can then be increased weekly by 500 mg (e.g. 1000 mg with dinner or 500 mg with dinner plus 500 mg with breakfast) based on blood sugar level. The maximum daily dose of metformin is 2500 mg.

The ADA does not recommend use of metformin in patients with hypertension, pre-eclampsia, or at risk for intrauterine growth restriction due to the potential for growth restriction or acidosis in the setting of placental insufficiency. However, American College of Obstetricians and Gynecologists (ACOG) and the Society for Maternal-Fetal Medicine do not give any such recommendation to avoid metformin in these situations.

Starting dose of glibenclamide (glyburide) is 2.5 to 5 mg once daily. Dose is then increased as needed to a maximum of 20 mg per day. Twice-daily dosing is often necessary to maintain glucose levels in the target range. Maternal hypoglycemia is the most common side effect.

Insulin Treatment

Regular insulin, insulin aspart, insulin lispro (U-100 and U-200), NPH, and insulin detemir all carry a pregnancy category B. For these insulins, the FDA has received sufficient human data allowing these to be considered low risk in pregnancy. Insulin glulisine, insulin degludec, and inhaled human insulin are all category C agents because there is no human data during pregnancy. Insulin glargine no longer has a pregnancy category, and its package inserts simply state that there are "no well-controlled clinical studies in pregnant women".

Estimation of Insulin Requirement during Pregnancy

Total insulin requirement per day

0.7 U/ kg, for 6 – 18 weeks

0.8 U/kg, 18 – 26 weeks

0.9 U/kg, 26 – 36 weeks

1 U/kg, 36 – 41 weeks

Note that the insulin requirement increases as the gestational age increases. The total insulin dose per day is based on gestational week and the woman's body weight. Twin gestations will approximately double the insulin requirement. In markedly obese patients, total required insulin may be in the range of 2–3 units/kg/day at term. Type 2 diabetes sometimes requires more insulin than type 1 diabetes due to insulin resistance.

It is better to start with a simple insulin regimen and then go on increasing the number of injections per day if the glucose targets are not met. Insulin pumps are not needed for majority of pregnant patients. Pregnant patients usually do not require admission to initiate insulin. However, if the patient needs to learn the technique of insulin, then admission may be considered.

Starting Insulin in Pregnancy

- Initially insulin can be started as a single dose in the morning. Human premix or analogue premix can be used for this purpose. A common practice is to begin human premix (30/70) at a dose of 10 to 15 units before breakfast.
- If postprandial glucose levels throughout the day remain high, dose is increased by 10 to 20 percent.
- If only the post-dinner glucose level remains elevated, then 6 to 10 units of short acting insulin (human insulin or analogue insulin) is added before dinner.
- If only the post-lunch glucose level remains elevated, then 6 to 10 units of short acting insulin (human insulin or analogue insulin) is added before lunch.
- If only the FBS is high (and PPBS values are normal), an intermediate-acting insulin (NPH) is given before bedtime but

before dinner is another option on an individualized basis; an initial dose of 0.2 unit/kg body weight is utilized. If it is being given before dinner, it can be combined with short acting insulin which is being given before dinner. For this purpose a premix insulin can be used before dinner or both insulins can be mixed before injection. A long-acting insulin analog (insulin glargine or detemir) may also be used instead of NPH.

- If only PPBS values are high (and FBS is normal), 6 to 10 units of rapid-acting insulin analogs (aspart or lispro) are given immediately before meals, and then adjusted as required.
- If both FBS and PPBS values are high, then it is preferable to start multiple daily injections per day.

Patient should monitor her blood glucose levels at home while on insulin therapy using glucometer. Ideally blood glucose should be checked at least 4 times daily. Once before breakfast (i.e. fasting glucose level) and at one or at two hours after the beginning of each meal. She should be taught about the symptoms of hypoglycemia (weakness, tingling sensation, diaphoresis, palpitations) and she should respond to it by first checking blood glucose. If the level is < 60 mg/dL, administer 10 to 20 g of a fast-acting carbohydrate snack immediately (half cup juice or 1 cup of skim milk or 5 to 6 hard candies; glucose tablets can also be used).

Blood glucose should be checked again 15 to 30 minutes after treatment. If the glucose remains <60 mg/dL, repeat treatment may be necessary. If low glucose values are encountered more than once at the same time of day, insulin doses are adjusted downward accordingly.

TIMING OF DELIVERY

Diabetes itself is not an indication for cesarean section or for delivery before 38 completed weeks of gestation. Continuation of pregnancy beyond 38 weeks increases the risk of fetal macrosomia, without reducing cesarean rates. So delivery at 38 weeks is recommended unless obstetric considerations dictate otherwise (ADA guidelines).

Management during Delivery

Whatever may be the type of diabetes (type 1 or type 2 or GDM), maintenance of good glycemic control during labor is essential to decrease the chances of fetal hypoxemia and neonatal hypoglycemia **(Fig. 10.1)**. During intrapartum period insulin requirement may become less due to the contracting uterus which utilizes glucose and also due to food restriction during labor. A reasonable target range for intrapartum glucose levels is 70 to 125 mg/dL. Various regimens have been suggested and tested in trials, including subcutaneous insulin, combined insulin glucose infusions or most commonly separate glucose and insulin infusions. Separate insulin and glucose infusion is the preferred regimen and works well in practice. Usually insulin infusion at the rate of 0.5–1 unit/hour is required. If the patient is being induced and is unlikely to be in active labor for several hours, the routine subcutaneous insulin dose can be given with her meals. A dose reduction of 20 to 30 percent may be necessary if the patient's blood glucose levels have been tightly controlled at home or if the patient is not eating adequately.

After food is restricted — as the patient enters active labor or when food becomes restricted, start dextrose-containing intravenous fluids (5 or 10 percent dextrose) and start an intravenous insulin infusion. Dextrose-containing fluids can be withheld if the blood glucose is ≥160 mg/dL. This will bring blood glucose into the target range (70 to 125 mg/dL) more rapidly. After the blood glucose declines below 160 mg/dL, the dextrose-containing fluids can be started. Patients who present with significant hyperglycemia (e.g. >200 mg/dL) may have an insulin infusion started in early labor, rather than waiting until active labor. Another option is to add a fixed dose of insulin to 5% dextrose solution. Add 6–8 units of regular insulin or analogue like lispro or aspart to 500 ml of 5% dextrose normal saline (DNS) according to the requirement of the patient **(Fig. 10.1)**. But note that if the patient's requirements are high it is advisable to start a separate insulin infusion with monitoring of the blood glucose every 1–2 h and to titrate the insulin infusion rate accordingly.

For those patients who are on intravenous insulin infusion blood glucose should be monitored every hour during active phase of labor and insulin adjusted accordingly. In patients on subcutaneous insulin or on no insulin during labor, blood glucose level can be monitored every two to four hours, depending on the stability of the blood glucose levels.

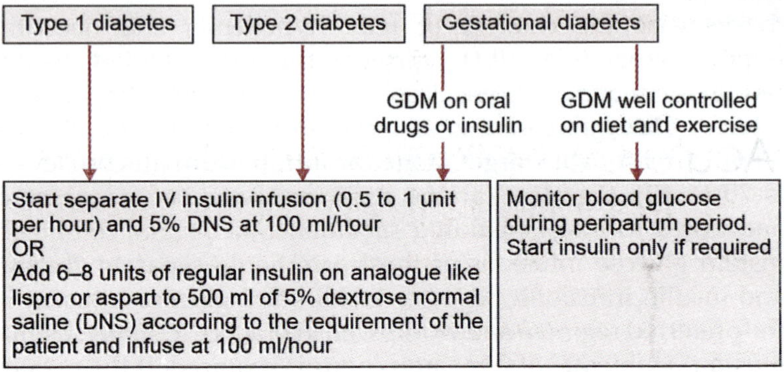

Fig. 10.1: Intrapartum management of diabetes

Postpartum

There is increased insulin sensitivity for a few days postpartum, hence, glucose levels should be monitored frequently, and insulin adjusted as required. For type 1 and type 2 diabetes patients, once the glucose is persistently >180 mg/dL, 90% of pre-pregnancy insulin dose can be prescribed and adjusted according to sugar levels. Do not aim for a very tight sugar control during the first 6 weeks of postpartum, as there would be disordered meal plan, disruptions of sleep, etc. owing to the stress of caring for the baby. Reasonable control of sugars is ok during this period. Women with gestational diabetes rarely require insulin in the postpartum period. As insulin resistance quickly resolves, so does the need for insulin. In patients who required insulin therapy during pregnancy, it is reasonable to check fasting and two-hour postprandial glucose levels before hospital discharge. Because women with gestational diabetes are at high risk for developing type 2 diabetes in the future, they should be tested for diabetes six weeks after delivery and yearly thereafter.

Chapter

11

Acute Complications of Diabetes Requiring Insulin Therapy

Diabetic ketoacidosis (DKA) and hyperosmolar hyperglycemic state (HHS) are the two most serious complications of diabetes, which can occur in both type 1 and type 2 diabetes. DKA is more common in type 1 DM and HHS is more common in type 2 DM. Mortality rate for DKA in experienced centers is less than 5% and for HHS around 15%.

Basic underlying mechanism of pathogenesis in both is relative or absolute deficiency of insulin and increase in counter regulatory hormones, which leads to increased hepatic and renal glucose production and decreased peripheral utilization, giving rise to hyperglycemia and increasing osmolality of ECF. In DKA, there is also increased release of free fatty acids into the circulation due to the same mechanisms as above and there is unrestrained hepatic fatty acid oxidation giving rise to ketone bodies (β-hydroxy butyric acid and acetoacetate) with resulting ketonemia and metabolic acidosis. This fatty acid breakdown is not seen in HHS.

The most common precipitating factor in the development of DKA or HHS is infection. Other causes include CVA, alcohol abuse, myocardial infarction, trauma, drugs, pancreatitis, discontinuation of insulin, etc. Intake of drugs that affect the carbohydrate metabolism, such as corticosterioids, thiazides and sympathomimetic drugs (e.g. dobutamine and terbutaline) may precipitate the development of HHS and DKA. Psychological disorders complicated by eating disorders like bulimia nervosa may also be a precipitating factor.

CLINICAL FEATURES

DKA can develop in less than 24 hours whereas HHS evolves more slowly over days or weeks. In both cases patient may give history of polyuria, polydypsia, polyphagia, weight loss, and vomiting. Nausea and vomiting are present in 50–80% of patients with DKA. History of pain abdomen may be there in DKA which may be due to DKA itself or a precipitating factor like appendicitis, pancreatitis, etc. Examination may reveal signs of dehydration like dry mucous membranes, loss of skin turgor, sunken eyes, tachycardia, hypotension, etc. in both DKA and HHS. Acidotic breathing (kussmal respirations) may be noted in DKA. Altered mental status may be present in both which may range from stupor to coma. Coma is more frequent in HHS. 25% of DKA patients may have coffee ground vomitus because of hemorrhagic gastritis. Even though infection may be the precipitating factor, patients may not have fever. Presence of hypothermia is a poor prognostic indicator.

Diagnostic Criteria for DKA and HHS (Table 11.1)

Table 11.1: DKA and HHS

Plasma Glucose (mg/dL)	350 to 500 (usually <800)	Frequently exceeds 1000 mg/dL
Fluid deficit	6 Litres	9 Litres
Arterial pH	<7.30	>7.30
Serum bicarbonate (mEq/L)	Usually <15	>15
Urine ketones	Positive	Absent or small
Serum ketones	Positive	Absent or small
Effective serum osmolality (mosm/kg)	Variable	>320
Anion gap	>10	Variable
Alteration in sensorium or mental obtundation	Alert (coma in severe cases)	Stupor/coma

Urine and serum ketones are measured by nitroroprusside reaction method
Effective serum osmolality = 2 [measured Na(mEq/l)] + glucose (mg/dL)/18
Anion gap (mEq/l) = (Na) – (Cl^- + HCO_3)

Differential Diagnosis

- *Starvation and alcoholic ketoacidosis* can be distinguished by clinical history and blood glucose values, which ranges from mildly elevated to rarely >250 mg/dL to hypoglycemia. The serum bicarbonate in starvation ketosis is usually not lower than 18 mEq/L.
- *Lactic acidosis*, history of metformin intake should be sought. Measurement of blood lactate levels will help.
- *CKD*: Clinical history will help. There is hyperchloremic acidosis rather than high anion gap acidosis.
- *Ingestion of salicylate, methanol, ethylene glycol and paraldelyde* can cause similar picture like DKA. Clinical history and measurement of serum salicylate, methanol will help. Presence of calcium oxalate and hippurate crystals in urine suggests ethylene glycol ingestion. Paraldehyde ingestion is suggested by strong odor in breath (characteristic odor).

MANAGEMENT OF ADULT PATIENTS WITH DKA

Principles of Treatment

- Correction of dehydration, hyperglycemia, and electrolyte imbalance.
- Identification and treatment of precipitating events.
- Frequent patient monitoring.

Quick Initial Assessment

Check airway and breathing first especially in patients with altered sensorium. Take focused history and do brief physical examination. Obtain arterial blood gases, TC, DC, ESR, urinalysis, blood glucose, blood urea, serum creatinine, serum electrolytes, chemistry profile, and an ECG. Order chest X-ray and cultures if necessary.

Inpatient vs Outpatient Treatment

Patients with mild DKA who are alert and taking fluids orally can be treated on OPD basis under observation. The ADA guidelines for admission are a plasma glucose concentration greater than 250 mg per dL with an arterial pH level below 7.30, a serum bicarbonate level of less than 15 mEq per L, and a moderate or greater level of ketones in the serum or urine. Patients with severe DKA require admission in the intensive care unit.

Fluid Replacement

Fluid replacement is the first priority while managing DKA and HHS. Fluid deficits are typically 100 mL per kg of body weight. Fluid replacement alone will lower blood glucose. Many studies have shown that during the first four hours of therapy for DKA, up to 80 percent of the decline in glucose concentration may be caused by fluid replacement. The effective serum osmolality ideally should not change more than three mOsm per hour during fluid replacement. The rate of initial isotonic saline infusion depends on the clinical state of the patient as follows.

- In patients with hypovolemic shock, isotonic saline should be infused as quickly as possible.
- In hypovolemic patients without shock (and without heart failure), isotonic saline is infused at a rate of 15 to 20 mL/kg lean body weight per hour (approximately 1000 mL/hour in an average-sized person) for the first couple of hours, with a maximum of <50 mL/kg in the first four hours.
- In euvolemic patients, isotonic saline is infused at a lower rate, guided by clinical assessment.

After the second or third hour, further fluid replacement should also take into account the sodium level. The "corrected" sodium concentration is calculated by adding 2 mEq/L to the plasma sodium concentration for each 100 mg increase in glucose level above normal. If the "corrected" serum sodium concentration is less than 135 mEq/L, isotonic saline should be continued at a rate of approximately 250 to 500 mL/hour. If sodium is normal or elevated, the IV fluid is generally switched to one-half isotonic saline at a rate of 250 to 500 mL/hour in order to provide more of electrolyte-free water.

When blood glucose approaches 200 mg/dL in DKA or 250 to 300 mg/dL in HHS, IV fluid is switched to dextrose in saline (DNS) and attempt is made to decrease the insulin infusion rate to 0.02 to 0.05 units/kg per hour. If possible, do not allow the serum glucose at this time to fall below 200 mg/dL in DKA or 250 to 300 mg/dL in HHS, because this may promote the development of cerebral edema.

Insulin Therapy

Unless the episode of DKA is mild, intravenous insulin infusion is the treatment of choice. In adult patients, once hypokalemia (K^+<3.3 mEq/L) is excluded, an intravenous bolus of regular insulin at 0.1 units/kg body wt, followed by a continuous infusion of regular insulin at a dose of 0.1 unit/kg/h (5 to 7 units/hr in adults), should be started. This initial insulin bolus is not recommended in pediatric patients as they may be very sensitive to insulin, instead a continuous insulin infusion of regular insulin at a dose of 0.1 unit/kg/h, may be started in these patients. Rapid acting insulin analogues (lispro, aspart, and glulisine) do not have any advantages over regular insulin when used as IV infusion. Any long-acting insulin should be withheld during DKA treatment. If the patient is on subcutaneous or intraperitoneal insulin pump, it should be stopped and the patient should be switched to an intravenous infusion. Aim for a decrease of plasma glucose concentration by 50 – 75 mg/dL/hour. If plasma glucose does not fall by 50 mg/dL from the initial value in the 1st hour, check hydration status; if necessary, the insulin infusion may be doubled every hour until a steady glucose decline between 50 and 75 mg/h is achieved (Fig. 11.1).

If infusion pump is not available, SC route may be used. Then the initial bolus is 0.4 units/kg (out of this half is given IV and half is given as SC).

Direct measurement of β-hydroxy butyrate (β-OHB) in the blood is the preferred method for monitoring DKA. The nitroprusside method only measures acetoacetic acid and acetone. However, β-OHB, the strongest and most prevalent acid in DKA is not measured by the nitroprusside method. During therapy, β-OHB is converted to acetoacetic acid, which may lead the clinician to believe that ketosis has worsened. Therefore, assessments of urinary or serum ketone levels by the nitroprusside method should not be used as an indicator of response to therapy. During therapy for DKA or HHS,

Regular inulin 0.1 U/kg as IV bolus

↓

0.1 U/kg/hour IV insulin infusion

↓

If serum blood glucose does not fall by 50–70 mg/dL in first hour

↓

Double insulin infusion hourly until glucose falls by 50–70 mg/dL

↓

When serum glucose reaches 200 mg/dL, continue insulin infusion at 0.02 to 0.05 units/kg per hour
OR
5–10 units every 2 hourly
Adjust to keep blood glucose between 150–200 mg/dL until metabolic control is achieved

Fig. 11.1: Insulin infusion in DKA

blood should be drawn every 2–4 h for determination of serum electrolytes, glucose, blood urea nitrogen, creatinine, osmolality, and venous pH (for DKA). Generally, repeat ABG studies are unnecessary; venous pH (which is usually 0.03 units lower than arterial pH) and anion gap can be used to monitor resolution of acidosis.

Criteria for resolution of DKA includes a glucose < 200 mg/dl, serum bicarbonate ≥ 18 mEq/L, and a venous pH of >7.3. Typical duration of therapy of DKA is usually 48 hours. Once DKA is resolved, if the patient is NPO, continue intravenous insulin and fluid replacement and supplement with subcutaneous regular insulin as needed every 4 h. In adult patients, this can be given in 5-unit increments for every 50 mg/dl for up to 20 units for blood glucose of ≥300 mg/dL. When the patient is able to eat, a multiple subcutaneous dose schedule should be started that uses a combination of short- or rapid-acting and intermediate- or long-acting insulin as needed to control plasma glucose. Continue intravenous insulin infusion for 1 to 2 hours after the subcutaneous regimen is begun to ensure adequate plasma insulin levels. Sudden discontinuation of intravenous insulin coupled with the delayed onset of subcutaneous insulin action may lead to loss of glycemic control; therefore, some overlap should occur in intravenous insulin therapy and initiation of the subcutaneous insulin regimen. Patients who were on insulin earlier may be given the same dose, which is further adjusted as necessary. In the newly diagnosed diabetic, the initial total daily insulin dose should be approx 0.5–1 unit 1 kg/day, divided into twice-daily mixed insulin regimen and adjusted as required. Newly detected type 2 diabetes patients may be discharged on oral antidiabetic agents and diet therapy.

Potassium Replacement

If K is <3.3 mEq, withhold insulin and give IV potassium chloride (KCl; 20 to 40 mEq/hour). This can be done by adding 20 to 40 mEq of KCL to each litre of saline. Hourly serum potassium measurement can be done until the serum potassium concentration above 3.3 mEq/L.

If K is between 3.3 and 5.3 mEq/L, IV KCl (20 to 30 mEq) is added to each liter of IV replacement fluid. Adjust potassium replacement to maintain the serum potassium concentration in the range of 4 to 5 mEq/L.

If K is ≥5.3 mEq/L, do not give any K, monitor hourly.

Bicarbonate Replacement

If pH is <6.9, give NaHCO3, 100 mEq diluted in 400 ml of distilled water, administered over 2 hours. If the serum potassium is less than 5.3 mEq/L, add 20 mEq of KCl.

The venous pH and bicarbonate concentration should be monitored every two hours, and bicarbonate doses can be repeated until the pH rises above 7.0.

Phosphate

Although the phosphate level is frequently low in patients with DKA, many studies have shown that routine phosphate replacement does not improve outcomes in DKA, and excessive replacement can lead to hypocalcemia. However, if severe hypophosphatemia occurs (serum phosphate below 1 mg/dL), especially if cardiac dysfunction, hemolytic anemia, and/or respiratory depression develop, phosphate replacement should be strongly considered. Phosphate can be given as potassium or sodium phosphate 20 to 30 mEq added to 1 L of IV fluid.

Magnesium

A serum deficit of 1 to 2 mEq per L of magnesium usually exists in DKA. DKA may alter the metabolism of magnesium. In addition, many patients with diabetes may be on diuretics which may lower magnesium levels. Symptoms of magnesium deficiency are difficult to recognize and overlap with symptoms caused by deficiencies of calcium, potassium, and sodium. Paresthesias, tremor, carpopedal spasm, agitation, cardiac arrhythmias and seizures are reported symptoms. Patients usually are symptomatic at serum levels of 1.2 mg per dL or lower. Consider magnesium replacement if the level is below normal i.e., less than 1.8 mg per dL and symptoms are present.

Use of Subcutaneous Route in DKA

In resource poor settings, or when ICU bed is not available, using S/C route of insulin administration for the management of DKA is comparable to IV insulin administration. Studies using S/C rapid acting insulins such as lispro and aspart have shown similar efficacy as IV route. Regular insulin can also be used S/C to treat DKA. Most of the studies have been done on mild to moderate DKA.

Initially 0.3 U/kg of regular insulin (or lispro or aspart) is given subcutaneously, followed by 0.1 U/kg insulin every hour or every 2 hours (0.2 units/kg) subcutaneously until blood glucose was <250 mg/dL. Then the insulin dose is decreased by half to 0.05, or 0.1 U/kg and administered every 1 or 2 hours until resolution of DKA.

MANAGEMENT OF ADULT PATIENTS WITH HHS

The principles of management of HHS are same as that of DKA with following changes.

Fluid deficit is more in HHS (average of 100–200 ml/kg, or 9 liters) than DKA; hence more fluids may be required. IV fluids should be changed to 5% dextrose with 0.45% saline when the blood glucose falls to 250 to 300 mg/dL. It is important to maintain serum glucose between 250 and 300 mg/dL till plasma osmolality is ≤315 mOsm/kg and patient is mentally alert. There is no role for bicarbonate therapy as pH is not affected in HHS.

Complications of DKA and HHS

- Hypoglycemia due to overzealous insulin therapy
- Hypokalemia due to insulin and bicarbonate therapy
- Cerebral edema — rare but frequently fatal complication of DKA, most common in children (0.7 – 1% DKA in children). It may also occur in HHS. Clinical features include decrease in the level of consciousness, lethargy, and headache. Rapid neurological deterioration may occur, with seizures, incontinence, pupillary changes, bradycardia, and respiratory arrest. Cerebral edema most likely happens because of rapid decline in plasma osmolality with treatment. It is minimized by gradual replacement of sodium and water (maximal reduction in osmolality 3 mOsm/kg H_2O/hour).
- ARDS can occur in DKA.

Chapter

12

Somogyi Phenomenon and Dawn Phenomenon

These two phenomenons may occur during insulin therapy. They have important clinical implications in the management of diabetes. It is important to recognize them and take appropriate corrective actions.

SOMOGYI PHENOMENON

It is also known as post-hypoglycemic hyperglycemia. Dr Michael Somogyi speculated (1930s) that insulin-induced hypoglycemia can produce hyperglycemia through counter-regulatory hormone responses. Excess insulin at night can produce unrecognized nocturnal hypoglycemia which can lead to morning hyperglycemia due to stimulation of secretion of counter regulatory hormones. The physician or patient may interpret this morning hyperglycemia as due to inadequate night dose of insulin and increase the night dose, further exacerbating the problem.

Defense against hypoglycemia involves counter regulatory hormones, which stimulate gluconeogenesis and glycogenolysis which restore the glucose levels in the blood. Counter-regulatory hormones include glucagon, epinephrine, cortisol and growth hormone. Glucagon acts on the liver to stimulate glycogenolysis and gluconeogenesis. Epinephrine increases the delivery of substrates from the periphery; decreases insulin release; stimulates glucagon release; inhibits glucose utilization by several tissues; and stimulates a warning system with sweating, anxiety, and tachycardia. Cortisol may aid in prolonged and severe cases of Somogyi phenomenon by blocking glucose utilization and stimulating hepatic glucose output. Growth hormone action is similar to cortisol.

Many studies have cast doubt on this mechanism of hypoglycemia stimulating counter-regulatory hormones leading to hyperglycemia. Some studies have shown that there is midnight hyperglycemia due to low insulin levels which continues as morning hyperglycemia rather than hypoglycemia stimulating hyperglycemia. Recently proposed mechanisms of morning hyperglycemia include nocturnal growth hormone secretion, hypoinsulinemia, and insulin resistance associated with metabolic syndrome.

Hypoinsulinemia (waning of the insulin dose), insulin resistance, and hypersensitivity to the effects of the counter-regulatory-hormones may play a role.

Causes

- Excess or ill-timed insulin
- Missed meals or snacks
- Inadvertent insulin administration

Frequency

There is very limited data on frequency of Somogyi phenomenon, but it is not very common. It is more common in type1 diabetes mellitus and less in type 2 diabetes mellitus. No age and sex predilection exists.

Diagnosing Somogyi Phenomenon

Patients present with morning hyperglycemia out of proportion to their usual glucose control. Nocturnal hypoglycemia is usually missed or asymptomatic. Somogyi phenomenon should be suspected in patients presenting with atypical hyperglycemia in the early morning that resists treatment with increasing insulin doses. Clinical signs, including weight gain, normal daytime blood sugar levels, and relatively low HbA1C should make one suspect Somogyi phenomenon. The most important thing in the diagnosis of Somogyi phenomenon is considering it in the causes of morning hyperglycemia.

Lab Studies

- Fasting blood sugar: The fasting blood sugar is expected to be inappropriately elevated due to hormonally induced rebound.
- Nocturnal (3–4 am) blood glucose: A glucose reading in the middle of the night will disclose hypoglycemia as a result of insulin therapy. This will establish the diagnosis.

Managing Somogyi Phenomenon

If nocturnal blood sugar is confirmatory or suspicion is high, reduce night or bedtime insulin. Giving nighttime intermediate insulin (NPH) at bedtime rather than before dinner may help. Substitution of night dose NPH with a longer acting preparation (glargine or detemir or degludec) will also help. Substitution of regular insulin with a fast-acting insulin analog, such as lispro or aspart, may be of some help. After the institution of these measures, continue glucose monitoring with special attention to hypoglycemia. Also, monitor weight and HbA1C. Educate patients about symptoms of hypoglycemia, proper insulin dose, timing of meals, and proper insulin administration.

DAWN PHENOMENON

It is due to early morning surge of growth hormone, which causes insulin resistance and early morning hyperglycemia. Dawn phenomenon is much more common than Somogyi phenomenon. Extended dawn phenomenon (persistence of hyperglycemia into the later morning hours) is also due to the same mechanism. In normal people without diabetes, there is small increase in insulin secretion before dawn, which suppresses hepatic glucose production and also counteracts the effect of growth hormone, thus preventing morning hyperglycemia.

It can be avoided by increasing the night dose of intermediate acting insulin (NPH) or basal insulin (glargine or detemir or degludec). If increasing night-time NPH causes midnight (3–4 am) hypoglycemia, then the timing of NPH injection can be shifted from dinnertime to bedtime. This will make the insulin peak to coincide with morning surge of growth hormone and controls hyperglycemia. Increasing the protein intake at night time rather than carbohydrates also helps to control dawn phenomenon.

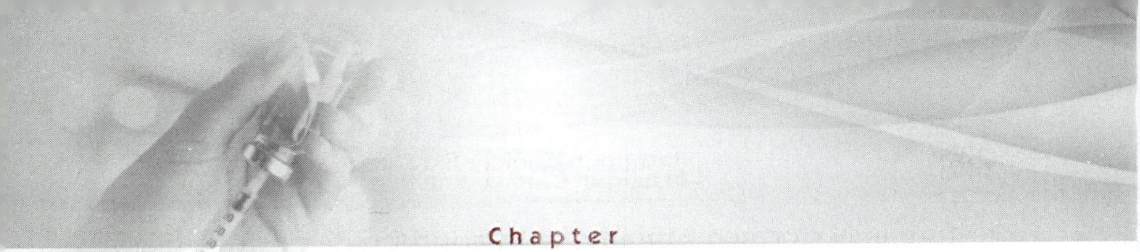

Chapter

13

Insulin Hypersensitivity (Allergy)

Insulin therapy can be complicated by the formation of anti-insulin antibodies. Earlier insulin preparations were more allergenic than the currently available insulins because of the use animal insulins and presence of impurities. Insulin hypersensitivity is less common with human insulin and insulin analogues. Hypersensitivity reactions may be caused by the insulin itself or by additives within the preparation (protamine and zinc). Though human insulin is less allergenic than animal insulin still it can induce production of antibodies due to the presence of impurities. Estimates of incidence of insulin hypersensitivity range from 0.1 to 7.1 percent of patients.

Hypersensitivity reactions can be immediate or delayed. Immediate reactions usually occur within one hour after an injection and often much more quickly. These reactions range from local erythema or a pruritic wheal at the injection site to systemic anaphylaxis. Immediate reactions are usually mediated by IgE and tend to worsen over time. Delayed reactions develop later than one hour and typically several hours to one or two days later. Common presentations include eczematous skin changes or induration or nodules at the sites of injection. Delayed reactions usually resolve spontaneously with time.

INVESTIGATING A CASE OF SUSPECTED INSULIN ALLERGY

First rule out improper injection technique, injection site infection because these can cause local redness and swelling which can be mistaken for hypersensitivity reactions. If these are ruled out then do a skin prick test to find out to which insulin or insulin component the patient is allergic. Prick testing is performed initially, with appropriate positive (e.g., histamine 10 mg/mL) and negative (e.g. saline 0.9 percent) controls. Insulins are applied undiluted for prick testing. If the initial readings of the prick tests are negative, then intradermal (intracutaneous) testing is done next, using insulin solutions that are diluted in saline 1:100. Most insulins are commercially available in a 100 unit/mL solution; a 1:100 dilution is equivalent to 1 unit/mL. Prior to undergoing skin testing for immediate reactions, patients must discontinue any antihistamines for a sufficient period of time (seven days for most agents).

Prick tests or intradermal tests are read after 15 minutes. A wheal with a diameter ≥3 mm is considered a positive reaction.

Management of Insulin Allergy

Almost all cases of insulin allergy can be treated successfully, and most can be resolved completely. The treatment depends on the type of allergy and the type of reaction. Local reactions usually lessen after 30 to 60 days of using the same insulin. During this waiting period, oral antihistamines can be prescribed to minimize the symptoms. The type of insulin may need to be changed to human insulin if the patient is reacting to animal insulin. If the insulin is changed from animal NPH to human NPH and still the symptoms continue, it could be due to protamine allergy and if this is a possibility try an insulin without protamine. If the patient is allergic to protamine, make sure this information appears prominently on the medical file-especially if the patient has heart problems. Protamine is commonly administered after cardiac surgery and could cause a severe reaction in an allergic patient. Protamine sulphate is also used sometimes after hemodialysis to neutralize heparin.

Allergy tests for different insulins and insulin components can indicate if a change to another insulin would solve the problem. Some people may be allergic to latex rubber, which can be mistaken for insulin allergy. This can happen due to latex in the syringe or the covering of insulin bottle. This possibility should always be kept in mind while investigating a case of insulin allergy. If the patient is allergic to latex, they should use syringes that contain no natural rubber and insulin bottles that do not have latex in the covering.

Allergic reactions can be lessened or avoided by using two injection sites and taking half the dose at each site. Another option is to inject low doses of steroids along with the insulin to prevent flare-ups. If these techniques do not work, consider other methods of insulin delivery such as using an insulin pump or insulin desensitization. Using CSSI can in many cases dramatically alleviate allergic reactions. It is not known exactly how pump therapy works to prevent local allergic reactions. It may be due to continuous exposure to small amounts of regular insulin round the clock which blunts the allergic response.

In patients with type 2 diabetes who are allergic to insulin, non-insulin therapies can be considered.

Insulin Desensitization

Insulin desensitization is a technique in which very small doses of insulin is injected initially and the dose is gradually increased every 15 to 30 minutes. Most of the people (up to 90%) can be desensitized by these methods. Desensitization should always be done with close monitoring and keeping resuscitative measures ready. A physician standby is also required. A sample desensitization protocol is given in **Table 13.1**.

Table 13.1: Sample insulin desensitization protocol

Day 1	0.0001, 0.001 and 0.005 IU every 15 to 30 minutes Then 0.01 IU every 30 minutes, achieving a total dose of 0.1 IU on day 1
Day 2	0.1 IU with an incremental dose of 0.05 IU every 30 minutes. Once the insulin dose reaches 0.5 IU, then incremental dose can be given at 0.1 IU every hour achieving a maximum dose of 1 IU of insulin per injection.
Day 3	Insulin is given at 1 IU, 2 IU and 3 IU at 30 minutes intervals (total of 6 units on day 3).
Day 4	Insulin is given at 4 IU tid and then gradually increased over the next few days.

Monitor glucose levels and allergic symptoms; prepare for emergency intervention.

In case of local allergic reactions, the last dose is repeated until no reaction occurs, and then the dose increases are continued. If a systemic reaction occurs, the reaction is treated as required. Once the symptoms have resolved, the protocol is resumed, starting with one-half of the dose that caused the reaction.

In the rare instances when desensitization does not work, steroids and antihistamines may have to be continued. The majority of cases tend to improve with simple treatments, such as switching to a different formulation of insulin, or waiting for the symptoms to resolve with time.

For persistent severe insulin allergy: divide the doses and inject into multiple sites; consider continuous subcutaneous insulin infusion with frequent changing of injection site; consider the addition of 1 μg dexamethasone per unit of insulin and/or systemic antihistamines.

Chapter

14

Insulin Resistance

Insulin resistance is a state in which a given concentration of insulin produces a less-than-expected biological effect. Usually patients requiring more than 1 unit/kg/day of insulin to maintain glycemic control are considered insulin resistant. Patients requiring greater than 200 units of exogenous insulin per day are considered severely insulin resistant. Most non-obese type 1 diabetic patients require 30–60 units of insulin per day, whether given IV or SC. Hence in a lean type 1 diabetic patient, insulin requirements of >1.5 U/kg/day are unusual and dosages >2 U/kg/day almost certainly indicate a significant underlying problem. Insulin resistance is a feature of type 2 DM, however, even type 1 diabetes also can have insulin resistance due to many reasons.

CAUSES OF INSULIN RESISTANCE

Obesity and sedentary lifestyle: Insulin sensitivity is impaired by obesity and/or lack of exercise.

Puberty: Increased GH secretion during puberty causes insulin resistance. For unknown reasons girls are more susceptible than boys.

Infections: Both acute and chronic infections (like tuberculosis) can cause insulin resistance.

Endocrine diseases: Like acromegaly, Cushing's syndrome, thyrotoxicosis and pheochromocytoma can cause increased secretion of counter regulatory hormones and hence increased insulin resistance.

Drugs: Such as glucocorticoids, thiazides, beta-agonists, etc. can cause insulin resistance. This is usually mild and can be easily overcome by increasing insulin dose.

Over insulinization: Over insulinization sometimes can lead to recurrent hypoglycemia, stimulation of counter regulatory measures and insulin resistance. A related entity called Mauriac syndrome has been described where over insulinization leads to excessive weight loss, hepatomegaly, and recurrent episodes of hypoglycemia. These features worsen if insulin dosage is increased and improve when dosage is reduced.

Defects in insulin pharmacokinetics or pharmacodynamics: This is extremely rare cause of insulin resistance. It is caused by defects in absorption of insulin from the site of injection especially at sites of lipodystrophy. Accelerated degradation of insulin also can cause increased insulin requirements.

Insulin binding Abs: Causes what is known as 'immune insulin resistance'. This was common with earlier impure insulins, especially bovine insulin. Insulin Abs can bind insulin, reducing its free circulating concentrations. Requirements may exceed 200 U/day. This problem has become less common now with the use of purer human insulin preparations.

Spontaneous development of insulin Abs to endogenous insulin can occur rarely in autoimmune disorders, plasma-cell dyscrasia, or in response to drugs (e.g. penicillamine, hydralazine, procainamide). These antibodies may interfere with the action of endogenous insulin and cause postprandial hyperglycemia and fasting hypoglycemia. With lymphoma or plasma cell dyscrasias, very high titres of high–affinity insulin antibodies may cause diabetes in previously nondiabetic individuals.

Insulin receptor and post receptor defects: can cause insulin resistance. Some of these types can be familial.

CAUSES OF APPARENT INSULIN RESISTANCE

Here actually there is no genuine insulin resistance. There are chances of physician interpreting it as insulin resistance if adequate details are not elicited from the patient.

Psychiatric and psychological problems: Can cause apparent increase in insulin resistance. Binge eating causes hyperglycemia and increased insulin requirements, which may be interpreted as insulin resistance.

Deliberate omission and under-dosing of insulin: Sometimes patients may not be taking the required dose and blood sugar values may be high. Physician may interpret this as inadequate insulin and may increase the dose unless proper history is elicited from the patient

Failure to understand or manage own diabetes: Noncompliance with diet and exercise, failure to monitor blood sugar values, incorrect techniques of insulin injection, use of an expired insulin bottle which has lost its potency, failure to visit the healthcare provider regularly etc may cause apparent insulin resistance.

INVESTIGATION OF A SUSPECTED CASE OF INSULIN RESISTANCE

Before doing more detailed investigations, the patient understanding of diabetes, compliance with diet and exercise, blood glucose monitoring, practical skills such as drawing insulin, checking the dose and injection techniques, etc. should be assessed. The expiry date and potency of insulin bottle or pen should be checked. If there is any doubt about the potency of insulin, new bottle should be used. Screening for infections (ESR, CRP, TC, DC, chest X-ray, urine microscopy, and culture) and endocrine diseases should be done as appropriate. Serum samples can be sent to specialist centers for determination of insulin Abs and insulin receptor Abs. If even after this the cause of insulin resistance remains undiagnosed then factitious insulin resistance should be considered. Rise in plasma insulin concentration and corresponding decrease in blood glucose should be determined after injecting test doses of insulin (0.1 U/kg) under standard conditions. The test injections should be given by doctor or nurse to ensure that the dose has been really injected.

Initial assessment: obtain detailed history from the patient as explained above. Elicit a detailed drug history. Examine the patient for Obesity (BMI, waist: hip ratio), pubertal status, signs of Cushing's disease, hypothyroidism, acromegaly, features of Mauriac syndrome. Look for any signs of chronic infections.

Look for the presence of acanthosis nigricans (association with insulin receptor defects).

Investigations: Screen for infections (ESR, chest X-ray, urine examination), endocrine diseases as appropriate. If the diagnosis is not made at this stage, admit the patient for further tests.

Further tests: Obtain 2nd hrly measurements of glucose and insulin levels for 48 hours while continuing current treatment. Doctors or nurses should give all insulin injections and not the patient or his caregivers. Also a formal psychosocial assessment of patient and family, screening for eating disorders can be done at this stage. If the cause of insulin resistance still remains unknown do gastric emptying studies, test for insulin and insulin receptor antibodies, and screen for drugs of abuse. If the cause is still undiagnosed do insulin challenge test.

Insulin Challenge Test

0.1 unit/kg of insulin is injected SC or IV. Obtain insulin and glucose levels every 30 minutes. Compare insulin and glucose profiles with normal ranges. A normal response indicates that the patient is noncompliant with the prescribed insulin regimen. If there is abnormal response, reconsider and investigate other diagnoses. Procedure for doing insulin challenge test to detect SC and IV insulin resistance is as follows

Preparation: Do not use long acting insulin previous day. Use IV insulin infusion (with normal saline) overnight to maintain glycemic control. Patient should fast overnight.

Subcutaneous Insulin Resistance Test

At about 9 am, discontinue insulin infusion to allow plasma glucose to rise to about 220–270 mg/dL.

Inject 0.1 U/kg of short acting insulin SC. Insulin should be given by a doctor from a new bottle of insulin. Take blood samples for glucose and free insulin levels, every 30 minutes for 4 hr. Patient should be monitored during the entire procedure. If blood glucose falls as expected, the test is stopped and it proves that the person does not have insulin resistance. If SC insulin resistance is demonstrated, proceed with intravenous test next day. Continue IV insulin infusion until next day to maintain reasonable glycemic control. If after IV injection blood glucose falls as expected, it means that the person has SC insulin resistance.

Intravenous Test

The next day, stop insulin infusion and allow the blood glucose to rise to 220–270 mg/dL. Inject 0.1 U/kg insulin IV as a bolus and take blood for glucose and insulin measurements as before.

Normal Results

SC: Maximum fall in plasma glucose should exceed 95 mg/dL
IV: Maximum fall in plasma glucose should exceed 60 mg/dL.
If not insulin resistance is confirmed.

MANAGEMENT OF A CASE OF INSULIN RESISTANCE

Once the cause for insulin resistance is known, treatment should be directed towards the underlying cause. Insulin dose can be increased while treating the underlying cause to maintain glycemic control. Sometimes changing over to an insulin analogue may solve the problem. The structural difference between insulin analogue and human insulin molecules may prevent insulin analogue from binding to the human insulin antibodies and consequently may be nonimmunogenic. Medications that reduce insulin resistance include metformin and thiazolidinediones.

Chapter

15

Non-Diabetic uses of Insulin

IN MYOCARDIAL INFARCTION

Diabetes mellitus insulin glucose infusion in acute myocardial infarction (DIGAMI) trial showed that treatment of acute MI patients especially those not in failure with high dose GIK (25% glucose, 50 IU/L of insulin; 80 mmol/L KCl) at 1.5 mL/kg/hour resulted in 30% relative risk reduction in death. However, many studies after this have shown conflicting results. At present time, GIK cannot be recommended as standard adjunctive treatment for MI. Many studies and a meta-analysis have shown that GIK infusion is cardioprotective in patients undergoing cardiac surgery.

In Hyperkalemia

Insulin causes potassium to shift into cells and temporarily lowers serum K levels, i.e. it buys time till more specific measures are instituted. Although glucose alone stimulates insulin release, a more rapid response occurs when exogenous insulin is given (with glucose to prevent hypoglycemia). Usually 10–20 units of regular insulin plus 100 ml of 25% or 50% glucose is administered intravenously as infusion. Hyperglycemic patients should not be given glucose. Plasma K will fall by 0.5 – 1.5 mEq/L in 15–30 minutes, and the effect will last for several hours.

In Peritoneal Dialysis

The fluid used for peritoneal dialysis contains varying concentration of dextrose (1.5%, 2.5%, 4.25% glucose) to create an osmotic gradient to facilitate filtration. This glucose may get absorbed from the peritoneal cavity and cause hyperglycemia. Adding insulin into the dialysis fluid can solve this problem but causes unpredictable absorption of insulin as the fluid is continuously being drained out. Hence subcutaneous regular insulin injections can be used to control hyperglycemia as appropriate.

To Test for Hypothalamic-pituitary-adrenal Axis

For this purpose insulin-induced hypoglycemia test (insulin tolerance test) is used. The rationale behind this test is that hypoglycemia induced by insulin is a sufficient stress to stimulate corticotropin-releasing hormone (CRH), corticotropin (ACTH), and therefore, cortisol secretion. Although this is a valid test of the hypothalamic-pituitary-adrenal response to stress, in most settings, the ACTH stimulation test provides nearly the same information, is much less difficult and less expensive to perform, and is without risk to the patient. Hence, insulin-induced hypoglycemia test is not performed frequently.

Chapter

16

Complications of Insulin Therapy

Just like any other therapeutic agent some side effects and complications can be seen with insulin therapy. These are as follows:

- Hypoglycemia
- Weight gain
- Insulin edema
- Lipodystrophy
  - Lipoatrophy
  - Lipohypertrophy
- Insulin allergy
- Anaphylaxis

HYPOGLYCEMIA

Hypoglycemia is more common with insulin therapy than oral therapy. Hypoglycemia is largely avoidable by frequent blood glucose monitoring and insulin dose adjustments. Patients should be educated about how to recognize hypoglycemia and how to take corrective actions. All the diabetic patients whether on oral drugs or insulin, should keep with them a readily available source of sugar (like sugar cubes or chocolates). Most hypoglycemia episodes will be mild and will not pose any significant problem if the corrective actions (like swallowing a sugar cube or chocolate) are taken immediately. Severe hypoglycemia episodes are defined as those requiring help from another person. If the hypoglycemia attack is severe, inj glucagon 1 mg IM can be given either at home or hospital. If at home this is the treatment of choice and patient should take oral glucose as soon as he is able to, otherwise he should be shifted to hospital. In the hospital 50 ml of 50% glucose intravenously will correct hypoglycemia. Patient may be at risk of developing further hypoglycemia and should be instructed to eat food. It is advisable to give 10% dextrose infusion for the next few hours.

Inj glucagon should be available at home of all diabetics and one or more family members should know how to inject it in emergencies. Children are often good at this as they have no apprehension or fear while injecting and they may be taught the technique of injection.

WEIGHT GAIN

In patients with severely uncontrolled diabetes, weight gain after starting insulin therapy is an inevitable consequence of the missing hormone's anabolic action and is due to restoration of fat and muscle bulk. Insulin therapy in both type 1 and type 2 diabetes may further increase body weight by ~ 1–1.5 kg and 2–3 kg, respectively, primarily as a result of reduced glycosuria. In type 2 diabetes metformin can help limit weight gain. Newer insulin analogues may be associated with less weight gain than conventional insulins. The importance of diet and physical exercise should be reinforced in all diabetic patients during routine follow up.

INSULIN EDEMA

This is a rare phenomenon seen at the start of insulin therapy in poorly controlled or previously untreated diabetic patients including those with ketoacidosis. Edema is due to acute sodium and water retention (a direct action of insulin on the renal tubule) after preceding long-term osmotic diuresis. It usually resolves spontaneously within a few days. For refractory insulin edema, ephedrine may be effective.

LIPODYSTROPHY

It can be of two types: Lipoatrophy and lipohypertrophy.

Lipoatrophy: This is caused by local reaction to insulin. Repeated injections into the same area and antigenic properties of insulin are blamed for this. Deposits of immune complexes at the site of injection followed by inflammation causes local wasting of subcutaneous fat, which may be seen as dimples in the area. Human insulin is less likely to cause this effect. Lipoatrophy does no harm except cosmetic disfigurement. When changed to newer purified insulins, lipoatrophy improves in 80% of patients within 3–6 months.

Lipohypertrophy: This is less common than lipoatrophy. Human insulin also has no benefit in reducing this effect. It is due to the accumulation of fat cells at the site of injection. The only preventive method is to change the site of insulin injections frequently. The painful lumps of lipohypertrophy can be mistaken for abcesses.

INSULIN ALLERGY

Insulin therapy in humans can be complicated by the formation of anti-insulin antibodies. Early insulin preparations were more immunogenic than the currently available insulins largely because of the presence of impurities in the earlier preparations. Though human insulin is less allergenic than animal insulin, it remains immunogenic.

Insulin allergy has been discussed in detail in Chapter 13 on insulin allergy.

Appendix I: Brand Names of Insulin Preparations Available in the Market

Brand Name	Manufacturer
Human Insulin (regular insulin)	
Human Actrapid	Novo Nordisk
Huminsulin R	Eli Lilly
Actrapid HM100 IU/mL Penfill cartridge	Novo Nordisk
Insugen-R, Actrapid	Biocon
Lupisulin-R	Lupin Ltd
Wosulin-R	Wockhardt Ltd
Recosulin-R (40 IU/mL, 10 mL vial)	Shreya
Insuman Rapid (100 IU/ mL)	Sanofi India Ltd
Insuman Rapid (40 IU/ mL)	Sanofi India Ltd
Insulin Lispro (rapid acting insulin)	
Humalog (100 IU/mL, 10 mL vial)	Cipla
Humalog (100 IU/mL 3mL cartridge)	Cipla
Eglucent Rapid 100 IU/mL solution for injection	Lupin
Humalog 100 IU/mL Kwikpen	
Insulin Aspart (rapid acting insulin)	
Novorapid (100 IU/mL, 10 mL vial)	Novo Nordisk
Fiasp FlexTouch pen (Fiasp is a modified form of aspart which is two times faster acting than aspart. Fiasp has niacinamide in it, which helps the body to absorb it faster) FlexTouch pens are easy to use disposable pens with a non-extending dose button that is specially designed to	Novo Nordisk

Contd...

Contd...

make it easier to inject. An audible 'click' sound lets you know that your full insulin dose has been delivered)	
Fiasp Penfill, 3 mL cartridge for pen, 100 IU/mL	Novo Nordisk
Novo Rapid Penfill (100 IU/mL, 3 mL cartridge for pen)	Novo Nordisk
Novo Rapid PumpCart, pre-filled insulin pump cartridge	Novo Nordisk
Insulin Glulisine (rapid acting insulin)	
Apidra 100 IU/mL	Sanofi Aventis
Pre-Mix Insulin (regular or rapid + intermediate acting)	
Mixtard 30: Soluble insulin 30% and isophane insulin 70%	Novo Nordisk
Mixtard 40: Soluble insulin 40% and isophane insulin 60%	Novo Nordisk
Mixtard 50: Soluble insulin 50% and isophane insulin 50%	Novo Nordisk
Wosulin 30/70: Suspension for injection 100 IU/mL	Wockhardt Ltd
Mixtard 30 HM 100 IU/mL Penfill	Novo Nordisk
Huminsulin 30/70 100 IU/mL Cartridge 3 mL	Eli Lilly
Mixtard 30 Suspension for injection 100 IU/mL	Novo Nordisk
NovoLog Mix 70/30 FlexPen	Novo Nordisk
NovoMix 30 (30% insulin aspart and 70% insulin aspart protamine)	Novo Nordisk
NovoMix 50 (50% insulin aspart and 50% insulin aspart protamine)	Novo Nordisk
NovoMix 70 (70% insulin aspart and 30% insulin aspart protamine)	Novo Nordisk
Humalog Mix 25 Kwikpen 100 IU/mL (Insulin Lispro 25% + Insulin Lispro Protamine 75%)	Eli Lilly
Humalog Mix 50 Kwikpen 100 IU/mL (Insulin Lispro 50% + Insulin Lispro Protamine 50%)	Eli Lilly
Insulin Glargine (basal insulin)	
Lantus (10 mL vial 100 IU/mL) Pen device	Sanofi India Ltd
Lantus SoloStar pen (100 IU/mL) Pen device	Sanofi India Ltd
Toujeo SoloStar pen (total units per pen = 450, maximum dose 80 units per injection)	Sanofi India Ltd
Toujeo max–SoloStar pen (total units per pen = 900, maximum dose 160 units per injection)	Sanofi India Ltd

Contd...

Contd...

Basalog One (disposable pen)	Biocon
Basugine (available as pen, cartridge, and 10 mL vial, all contain 100 IU insulin per mL)	Lupin Ltd
Glaritus (available as pen, cartridge, and 10 mL vial, all contain 100 IU insulin per mL)	Wockhardt Ltd
Glarzen (disposable pen)	Wockhardt Ltd
Basaglar (available as pen and 3 mL cartridge)	Cipla Ltd
Insulin Degludec (basal insulin)	
Tresiba 100 IU/mL Flextouch pen	Novo Nordisk
Tresiba 100 Units/mL Penfill	Novo Nordisk
Ryzodeg 100 IU/mL Flextouch pen (70% degludec + 30% aspart)	Novo Nordisk
Insulin Detemir (basal insulin)	
Levemir Flexpen (100 IU/mL)	Novo Nordisk

Insulin Pens	
NovoPen 4	It encompasses audible end of dose click reassuring dose delivery for an accurate insulin delivery
NovoPen 5	It has additional memory function and records time and dose volume since last injection
NovoPen Echo	The NovoPen Echo® comes with memory function and has fine-tuned half unit increment dosing
FlexPen	FlexPen® is pre-filled with insulin or GLP–1 Less force during injection compared to SoloSTAR® and KwikPen® Colour-coded pens make identification easy
Flex Touch	Non-extending dose button and low injection force make the injection easier to give End-of-dose click and patient confidence in accurate dose delivery
NovoPen 6 and NovoPen Echo Plus	Record time and date of all injected doses as well as the number of units dosed

Appendix II: Carbohydrate Content of Foods

The carbohydrate amounts listed here are estimates. These tables will help you in further fine tuning insulin adjustments especially when unexpected foods are eaten during functions, etc. Check the food label for the accurate amount of carbohydrate in that product.

MEASUREMENT KEY

1 tsp = 5 mL

3 tsp = 1 tb sp (15 mL)

½ cup = 4 ounces = 120 mL

4 tb sp = ¼ cup (60 mL)

1 cup = 8 ounces = 240 mL

5 1/3 tb sp = 1/3 cup

2 cup = 1 pint = 480 mL

Amount of starches/fruits that equal 15 grams carbohydrate

Starches	***Serving size***
Beans, cooked, dried, canned	1/3 cup
Bread, white, whole wheat, rye	1 slice (1 oz)
Corn, cooked	1/2 cup
Crackers	4 – 6
Hamburger bun	1/2 bun
Popcorn	3 cups
Pasta, cooked	½ cup
Peas, cooked	½ cup
Potato, baked	1 small (3 oz)

Contd...

Contd...

Potato, mashed	½ cup
Rice, cooked	1/3 cup
Tortilla medium	1
Fruits	
Apple, Small	1 (4 oz)
Applesauce, unsweetened	½ cup
Banana	1 small banana or ½ large
Blueberries	¾ cup
Canned fruit, light or juice packed	½ cup
Cantaloupe, melon	1 cup cubed
Cherries, sweet, fresh	1 2 (3 oz)
Fruit juice	½ cup (4 oz)
Grapefruit, medium	½
Grapes, small	17
Pear, large, fresh	1 (6 ½ oz)
Raisins	2 tb sp
Strawberries	1¼ cup whole berries
Watermelon	1¼ cup cubes

Other carbohydrates

Food	***Serving Size***	***Carbohydrate in gms***
Milk (skim, 1%, 2%, whole	1 cup (8 oz)	12 gm
Cake, unfrosted	2″ square	15 gm
Cake, frosted	2″ square	30 gm
Chicken noodle soap	1 cup (8 oz)	15 gm
Cookie (sandwich or chocolate chip)	2 cookies	15 gm
Food	***Serving Size***	***Carbohydrate in gms***
Cookie, medium (homemade)	1 cookie	15 gm
Cupcake, frosted	1 small	30 gm

Contd...

Contd...

Food	*Serving Size*	*Carbohydrate in gms*
Doughnut, plain cake	1 medium (1.5 oz)	20 gm
Doughnut, glazed	3¾ in. (2 oz)	30 gm
French fries, thin	20–25	30 gm
Ice cream (regular, light, fat free)	½ cup	20 gm
Jam or jelly, regular	1 tb sp	15 gm
Macaroni and cheese	1 cup (8 oz)	30 gm
Noodle casserole	1 cup (8 oz)	30 gm
Pie, fruit, 2 crusts	1/ 6 pie	45 gm
Potato chips	12–18 (1 oz)	15 gm
Pizza	1 slice (1/4 of 10″)	30 gm
Pudding, regular	½ cup (4 oz)	25 gm
Tomato soup (made with water)	1 cup (8 oz)	15 gm
Yogurt, light	1 cup (6 – 8 oz)	15 gm

Carbohydrate content of some sugar rich foods

Food item	*Serving quantity*	*Carbohydrate in gm*
Beverages		
Cola drinks	12 oz can	50
Rootbeer	12 oz can	35
7-up	12 oz can	45
Grape, orange, apple juice	6 oz can	25
Dairy Products		
Sherbet	1 scoop	45
Ice cream cone	1 scoop	17
Chocolate milk shake	10 oz glass	55
Milk	8 oz glass	15
Chocolate milk	8 oz glass	52

Contd...

Contd...

Cakes and Cookies		
Chocolate cake, plain	4 oz piece	30
Chocolate cake,	4 oz piece	50
Sugar cookie	1	7
Oatmeal cookie	1	10
Donut, plain	1	20
Donut, glazed	1	30
Desserts		
Pastry	4 oz piece	20
Apple pie	1 slice	35
Berry pie	1 slice	50
Chocolate pudding	½ cup	20
Candies		
Chocolate candy bar	1 ½ oz	12
Chewing gum	1 stick	2
Hard candy	1 oz	25
Chocolate crème	1 piece	10
Miscellaneous		
Jelly	1 tb sp	15
Strawberry jam	1 tb sp	15
Sugar	1 tb sp	15
Honey	1 tb sp	15
Chocolate sauce	1 tb sp	15

Index